Nurse-Led Health Clinics

Tine Hansen-Turton, MGA, JD, FCPP, FAAN, is a social entrepreneur who has started several national and global social and public innovations in the health and human services sector. For the past two decades she has been instrumental in leading a movement of nurse-led primary health care, positioning advanced practice nurses and nurse practitioners as primary health care providers. She is currently the chief strategy officer of Public Health Management Corporation (PHMC), where she oversees and leads corporate strategy, development, and operations for a public health institute. She serves as CEO of the National Nursing Centers Consortium, a nonprofit organization supporting the growth and development of over 500 nurse-led health centers, serving more than 2.5 million vulnerable people across the country. Additionally, she serves as the founding executive director for the Convenient Care Association, the U.S.-based trade association of the private-sector retail clinic industry. She is co-author of numerous publications including but not limited to *Partnerships for Health and Human Service Nonprofits; Social Innovation and Impact in Nonprofit Leadership; Convenient Care Clinics: The Essential Guide for Clinicians, Managers, and Educators; Community and Nurse-Managed Health Centers: Getting Them Started and Keeping Them Going;* and *Nurse-Managed Wellness Centers: Developing and Maintaining Your Center.* In 2009 she cofounded *Philadelphia Social Innovations Journal* (PSIJ), an online publication that brings a focus to social innovators and their nonprofit organizations, foundations, and social sector businesses. Following the creation of PSIJ, she cofounded the Philadelphia Social Innovations Lab to serve as a hub to test new social models which she now teaches as an adjunct professor at University of Pennsylvania, Fels Institute of Government.

Susan Sherman, MA, RN, has served as president and CEO of the Independence Foundation since 1996. The Independence Foundation, a private philanthropy dedicated to supporting programs in Philadelphia and surrounding Pennsylvania counties that provide services to people who ordinarily do not have access to them, has four specific areas of funding: culture and arts; health and human services; nurse-managed primary health care; and public interest legal aid. Ms. Sherman is a member of the board of directors of the Public Health Management Corporation (PHMC), Project H.O.M.E., and the Academy of Vocal Arts, and was chairperson of the Philadelphia Award Committee. She serves on the advisory committees of the American Academy of Nursing, *Philadelphia Social Innovations Journal,* the Metropolitan AIDS Neighborhood Nutrition Alliance, Students Run Philly Style, and Meds & Eds Alliance. She also serves on the Eisenhower Fellowships Philadelphia International Leadership Initiative Steering Committee, the Pennsylvania Action Coalition Steering Committee, and the Pennsylvania Bar Association Judicial Evaluation Commission. She is a fellow of the American Academy of Nursing and the College of Physicians of Philadelphia.

Eunice S. King, PhD, RN, is a senior program officer and director of research and evaluation for the Independence Foundation, where she has overseen the foundation's grant making under the nurse-managed health care initiative. In addition, she is the program evaluation consultant to the National League for Nursing's Advancing Care Excellence for Seniors (ACES) program, a partnership between the National League for

Nursing and Community College of Philadelphia. Prior to joining the Independence Foundation, Dr. King was associate dean for research in the MCP Hahnemann School of Nursing at Drexel University, where she taught graduate courses in research and studied issues of medication adherence among individuals living with HIV and AIDS. Upon completion of her PhD studies, she joined the behavioral research staff of the Fox Chase Cancer Center Division of Population Science, where she conducted National Cancer Institute–funded studies that developed and tested strategies to promote mammography use among women, and a Pennsylvania Department of Health–funded study to encourage smoking cessation among pregnant women. Earlier in her career, Dr. King was a psychiatric nurse clinical specialist in a variety of health care settings, including an acute care psychiatric hospital, a community mental health clinic, and a general hospital. In addition, she held a faculty position at the Villanova University College of Nursing and was an independent psychiatric nursing consultant.

Nurse-Led Health Clinics

Operations, Policy, and Opportunities

Tine Hansen-Turton, MGA, JD, FCPP, FAAN
Susan Sherman, MA, RN
Eunice S. King, PhD, RN

Editors

SPRINGER PUBLISHING COMPANY

NEW YORK

Springer Publishing Company, LLC
11 West 42nd Street
New York, NY 10036
www.springerpub.com

Acquisitions Editor: Joseph Morita
Production Editor: Kris Parrish
Composition: Exeter Premedia Services Private Ltd.

ISBN: 978-0-8261-2802-7
e-book ISBN: 978-0-8261-2803-4

15 16 17 18 / 5 4 3 2 1

The author and the publisher of this Work have made every effort to use sources believed to be reliable to provide information that is accurate and compatible with the standards generally accepted at the time of publication. Because medical science is continually advancing, our knowledge base continues to expand. Therefore, as new information becomes available, changes in procedures become necessary. We recommend that the reader always consult current research and specific institutional policies before performing any clinical procedure. The author and publisher shall not be liable for any special, consequential, or exemplary damages resulting, in whole or in part, from the readers' use of, or reliance on, the information contained in this book. The publisher has no responsibility for the persistence or accuracy of URLs for external or third-party Internet websites referred to in this publication and does not guarantee that any content on such websites is, or will remain, accurate or appropriate.

Library of Congress Cataloging-in-Publication Data

Nurse-led health clinics : operations, policy, and opportunities / [edited by] Tine Hansen-Turton, Susan Sherman, Eunice S. King.
　　p. ; cm.
Includes bibliographical references and index.
ISBN 978-0-8261-2802-7 — ISBN 978-0-8261-2803-4 (e-book)
I. Hansen-Turton, Tine, editor.　II. Sherman, Susan, editor.　III. King, Eunice S., editor.
[DNLM: 1. Nurse's Practice Patterns.　2. Community Health Centers—organization & administration. 3. Community Health Nursing—organization & administration.　4. Organizational Case Studies.　5. Primary Health Care—organization & administration. WY 105]
RT98
362.12068—dc23

2014045557

Printed in the United States of America by McNaughton & Gunn

This book is dedicated to Lee Ford, the mother of nurse practitioners; Phyllis Beck, the chair of the Independence Foundation board of directors and longtime champion of nurse-managed health clinics; and Andrea Mengel, for her leadership on the Independence Foundation board of directors and her passion for the health-promoting work conducted by nurse-managed health clinics.

In addition, co-authors Tine Hansen-Turton and Eunice S. King dedicate this book to their co-author, colleague, and mentor, Susan Sherman, the mother of nurse-managed health clinics.

Contents

Contributors

Geraldine Bednash, PhD, RN, FAAN
Former Chief Executive Officer
American Association of Colleges of Nursing
Arlington, Virginia

Sally Coates, MSW, LCSW
Senior Director
Senior House Calls
Lubbock, Texas

M. Christina R. Esperat, PhD, RN, FAAN
Professor and Associate Dean
Texas Tech University Health Science Center School of Nursing
Lubbock, Texas

Kathryn Fiandt, PhD, FNP-BC, FAANP, FAAN
Integral Nursing Associates
Omaha, Nebraska

Loretta Ford, RN, PNP, EdD, FAAN, FAANP
Dean and Professor Emerita
University of Rochester School of Nursing
Rochester, New York

Patricia Gerrity, PhD, RN, FAAN
Associate Dean for Community Programs and Director
    of 11th Street Family Health Services
Drexel University College of Nursing and Health Professions
Philadelphia, Pennsylvania

Susan B. Hassmiller, PhD, RN, FAAN
Senior Advisor for Nursing & Director, Future of Nursing: Campaign for Action
Robert Wood Johnson Foundation
Princeton, New Jersey

Sarah Hexem, JD
National Nursing Centers Consortium
Philadelphia, Pennsylvania

Frances Hughes, MA, DNurs, RN, ONZM
Chief Nursing and Midwifery Officer
Nursing and Midwifery Office
Department of Health
Queensland Government Level 1
Queensland, Australia

Maureen E. Leonardo, MN, CRNP, CNE, FNP-BC
Clinical Associate Professor
Duquesne University School of Nursing
Pitcairn, Pennsylvania

Linda McMurry, DNP, RN, NEA-BC
Larry Combest Center
Texas Tech University Health Science Center School of Nursing
Lubbock, Texas

Andrea Mengel, PhD, RN
Independence Foundation Chair in Nursing
Community College of Philadelphia
Philadelphia, Pennsylvania

Mary Ellen T. Miller, PhD, RN
Assistant Professor
DeSales University Department of Nursing and Health
Conshohocken, Pennsylvania

Donald B. Parks, MD, FACP
Associate Professor of Community Medicine
Temple University School of Medicine
Philadelphia, Pennsylvania

Bonita Ann Pilon, PhD, RN-BC, FAAN
Senior Associate Dean
Vanderbilt University School of Nursing
Nashville, Tennessee

Lenore K. Resick, PhD, CRNP, FNP-BC, FAANP
Clinical Professor; Noble J. Dick Endowed Chair in Community Outreach; Executive
    Director, Community-Based Health & Wellness Center for Older Adults; Director,
    Family Nurse Program
Duquesne University School of Nursing
Emlenton, Pennsylvania

Sarah Rosenberg, JD
Membership & Development Director for the National Nursing Centers Consortium
    and the Convenient Care Association
Philadelphia, Pennsylvania

Nancy L. Rothman, EdD, MSN, MEd, RN
Professor of Urban Community Nursing
Temple University
Philadelphia, Pennsylvania

Sandra Festa Ryan, MSN, RN, CPNP, FCPP, FAANP, FAAN
Chief Clinical Officer
CareCam Health Systems
West Conshohocken, Pennsylvania

M. Elaine Tagliareni, EdD, RN, CNE, FAAN
Chief Program Officer
National League for Nursing
Washington, DC

Donna L. Torrisi, MSN, FAA
Network Executive Director
Family Practice & Counseling Network
Philadelphia, Pennsylvania

Jessie Torrisi, MS
Columbia University School of Journalism
New York, New York

Brian Valdez, JD
Policy and Development Specialist
National Nursing Centers Consortium
Philadelphia, Pennsylvania

Jamie M. Ware, JD, MSW
National Nursing Centers Consortium and Convenient Care Association
Philadelphia, Pennsylvania

Foreword

I believe that the entry of nurse practitioners (NPs) first into nurse-managed health clinic settings in the 1990s and then into convenient care (retail) clinic settings in the early 2000s was the most innovative, creative, and courageous effort to address the community health needs of surrounding populations ever undertaken. These NP-led clinics get an "A" on every score: accessibility, accountability (quality), and affordability, with the further benefits of availability, acceptability, and affability. Furthermore, the clinics have data to prove it. Early, sophisticated electronic patient data collection systems afforded a broad base for planning, executing, and evaluating NP practices and patient needs, desires, and demands.

None of this would have been possible without the expert NP leadership exemplified by Sandra Ryan, Donna Torrisi, and others, as well as by trade associations like the National Nursing Centers Consortium and the Convenient Care Association, both of which pushed for positive policy changes in state capitals and in Congress. These nursing leaders and leaders of the focused trade organizations brought professional nursing values; high standards for the practice, recruitment, and guidance of staff; enthusiasm and energy; and the amazing ability to work successfully within the complexities of the corporate world. These nursing leaders and associations bore the brunt of the challenges, mainly from organized medicine, of introducing the community-based, nurse-led, convenient care setting with the skills of participation, negotiation, decision making, and change theory, plus their intelligence, street smarts, staff support, and chutzpah.

The nurse-led clinic innovation and movement also introduced something very important to the current costly sector of sick care: prevention and health promotion. NPs are known for their blended skills of case finding, educating patients in health and illness self-management, and opening the gates to what could be the future of health care in this nation…moving from a sick care model of primary care to primary *health* care.

The data on the spread of nurse-led services, the millions of patients served, and the high level of patient acceptance and satisfaction position nurse-led care—whether in community-based nurse-managed health clinics or convenient care clinics—to fit well into the health care reform legislation to improve 21st century health care!

Fond regards, Lee (the mother of nurse practitioners)
(Loretta Ford, RN, PNP, EdD, FAAN, FAANP)
Dean and Professor Emerita
University of Rochester School of Nursing

Foreword

We are in an exciting time in the history of health care and nursing. The demand for health care services and the need for innovation and a strong nursing presence to meet patient needs has never been greater.

Nurse practitioners and nurse-led clinics and operations have been breaking new ground and are helping to meet the needs of patients nationally and globally! With over 1,600 nurse practitioner convenient care (retail) clinics, dozens of university nurse practice centers, and hundreds of community-based health care centers nationally, patients are receiving care by nurse practitioners in every community across our country.

It is more important than ever that these models of care delivery continue to succeed and meet the needs of the patients they are there to serve. In order to do that, nursing leaders must keep up with the latest research and be ready and willing to innovate, negotiate, communicate, and change themselves and the system to meet the needs of the patient. The use of technology will continue to advance and change the way we are doing business today. As nursing leaders, we must embrace the use of technology and look for innovative ways to keep the patient at the center of what we do. Patients will soon be receiving real-time information on their biological functioning through the use of sensor technology, and we must be ready to help them decide what they want to do with the information and to continue to be their trusted resources for guidance.

Health care is increasingly becoming driven by the patient, and the patient is becoming an active, informed player in this evolving, ever-changing sport. In the past, the provider–patient relationship was a one-way street: The health care provider made the diagnosis, engaged the patient in the health plan, and sent the patient out to execute the plan. Today, with shifts in the health care landscape in the way that performance and payment will be measured, and with innovations in technology and information readily available to patients, there has been an increasing demand for this relationship to be more of a two-way communication, with patients who are more educated, empowered, and engaged in their personal health.

As a nursing leader, I say to you: Our time is now! We must be at the table, we must be change agents who are seen as forward-leaning innovators in health care delivery, and we must always remain committed to putting our patients at the center of everything we do. Nursing is an honorable, knowledgeable profession that has contributed immensely to the health care system today. Let us remain strong, focused, and unwavering in our commitment to quality, affordable, convenient health care for all.

Sandra Festa Ryan, MSN, RN, CPNP, FCPP, FAANP, FAAN
Robert Wood Johnson Executive Nurse Fellow
Chief Clinical Officer, CareCam Health Systems
Past Chief NP Officer, Take Care Health Systems, Walgreens

Preface

We are pleased to present you with *Nurse-Led Health Clinics: Operations, Policy, and Opportunities*. In this book, we provide a historical perspective on nurse-managed health centers (NMHCs); include chapters on the practical aspects of starting and operating NMHCs, combined with case studies that illustrate the challenges, lessons learned, and successes of NMHCs; and conclude with an assessment of the current status of NMHCs and a vision for their future. It has been an honor and privilege to be part of such an incredible health care movement during the past 25 years and to help shape it into what it has become today. Nurse-managed health clinics represent a paradigm shift in health care, and we did not want their history to be left untold. The story holds many lessons. Nurse-managed health clinics have not only been a global policy and practice game changer for nursing and the role of nurse practitioners, but have also given birth to many other nurse-led models like retail clinics and school-based health clinics. The influence of NMHCs on the delivery of health care will only continue to evolve in decades to come.

We want to thank the thousands of nurses and non-nurses who have been passionate about this model of care and whose passion and commitment have inspired others. They laid the groundwork for the movement and had the vision for providing nurse-led quality, community-based care that is accessible and affordable to all. In particular, we wish to acknowledge the vital contributions of two organizations: the Independence Foundation and the National Nursing Centers Consortium (NNCC). The strategic work of the members, board, and staff leadership of the NNCC (www.nncc.us), whose mission is to advance nurse-led care globally, has effected changes in many health policies that have strengthened the viability of NMHCs and other nurse-led models of care. Since 1994, the board of the Independence Foundation has designated nurse-managed health care as one of its funding priorities and has supported NNCC and nurse-managed health clinics in the Philadelphia region for two decades. In 1996, NNCC and the Independence Foundation set out on a mission to put nurse-managed health clinics and nurse-led care on the global map and, as is evidenced by the book, their mission has been a success.

Tine Hansen-Turton
Susan Sherman
Eunice S. King

Introduction

Over a century ago, on the Lower East Side of New York City, a young New York Hospital nursing graduate named Lillian Wald was teaching immigrant women about home care and hygiene when a young child, the daughter of one of Wald's students, entered the classroom in tears. She told Wald that her mother was sick. Wald followed the child to her apartment, where a woman lay in a filthy, blood-soaked bed. The child's mother had given birth 2 days earlier and was hemorrhaging. Wald treated the woman, cleaned the room, and comforted the family.

That event compelled her to start the Henry Street Settlement, where she and her nursing colleagues dedicated their lives to caring for some of society's most vulnerable. They not only treated their community's health needs but also sought to improve where their neighbors lived, worked, and played. They offered social services and instruction in everything from music to English. In doing so, they became the first public health nurses in the country. They fearlessly focused on the needs of the poor, the aged, those suffering from social injustice, and those living in areas without access to adequate health care facilities.

In the years since Wald founded Henry Street, the nursing profession has continued to offer innovative solutions to meet the needs of patients, families, and communities. The challenges may differ, but the impetus that drove Wald to start Henry Street remains the same: to provide compassionate care to the most vulnerable and to improve health and health care for all. As our country undergoes rapid health care transformation, driven by an aging and sicker population, rapid technological innovation, persistent health care disparities, and skyrocketing costs, nurse leaders are devising solutions every day in communities large and small to improve health and health care for all.

Health care models increasingly rely on nurses to drive success. Nurses serve in clinical leadership and care coordinator roles. Certified nurse midwives offer pre- and postnatal care and assist with labor and delivery with little technological intervention at birthing centers. Advanced practice registered nurses provide a full range of health care services at nurse-managed health clinics, including primary care, health promotion, disease prevention, and behavioral health care to residents of underserved communities. And nurse practitioners at convenient care clinics improve access to care and save costs by enabling people with minor ailments to get treated in their communities rather than in the emergency room.

These innovative, nurse-managed solutions were featured in the Institute of Medicine's (IOM's) landmark report *The Future of Nursing: Leading Change, Advancing Health*, which offers a blueprint for how our country can improve health through nursing. The Robert Wood Johnson Foundation, the nation's largest philanthropy devoted to improving health and health care, and AARP, the nation's largest consumer organization, realized the potential of the IOM recommendations for improving our nation's health. That is why we launched The Future of Nursing: Campaign for Action, a 50-state initiative to advance the IOM recommendations and improve health and health care. The campaign seeks to promote practice and leadership, strengthen nursing education, foster interprofessional collaboration, and improve workforce diversity.

Up to 25 million Americans gained access to health insurance in 2014 under the Affordable Care Act, and our country needs to do everything it can to ensure that practitioners will be available to see these newly insured individuals when they need one. Nurse practitioners and nurse-managed health clinics can, without question, dramatically expand access to primary and preventive health care throughout the United States. Nursing's time is now.

Nurse-Led Health Clinics: Operations, Policy, and Opportunities is required reading for clinicians, nursing leaders, nurse-managed and convenient care clinic operators, managed care organizations, and physician organizations to fully understand the potential of nurse-managed clinics in the future of health care. It is my hope that many of the readers of this book will be inspired to open their own nurse-managed clinics and play an instrumental role in the future of health care, just as Lillian Wald did over a century ago.

Susan B. Hassmiller, PhD, RN, FAAN
Senior Advisor for Nursing, and Director, Campaign for Action
The Robert Wood Johnson Foundation

Introducing Nurse-Managed Models

Tine Hansen-Turton

Nurse-led models of care are dynamic health care innovations that provide accessible, affordable, high-quality, patient-centered care that integrates the mind and body, aims at high patient satisfaction, and produces outcomes that are as good as and often better than the care provided by MDs in traditional primary care clinical settings. Throughout this book, the terms *nurse-led care*, *nurse-managed health center*, *nurse-managed health clinic*, *nurse-led center*, and *nurse-practice arrangements* are used interchangeably. However, all terms should be interpreted as corresponding to the definition provided by the Patient Protection and Affordable Care Act (ACA). According to Section 5208 of the ACA, a nurse-managed health center (NMHC) is defined as "a nurse practice arrangement, managed by advanced practice nurses, that provides primary care or wellness services to underserved or vulnerable populations and that is associated with a school, college, university or department of nursing, federally qualified health center, or independent nonprofit health or social services agency" (42 U.S.C. § 330A–1) (Patient Protection and Affordable Care Act, 2010).

Section I opens with an introduction to the NMHC concept, including an overview of the history of NMHCs and a thorough discussion of what it will take for those who are interested in pursuing an NMHC to build a successful practice. Subsequently, a number of renowned practitioners and nursing leaders in the field contribute insights on specific aspects of NMHC care, such as practice sustainability, quality and safety, and behavioral health. Readers will acquire a very thorough grounding in NMHC operations and will find the material in this section to be a valuable guide to establishing a successful nurse-managed clinical practice.

REFERENCE

Patient Protection and Affordable Care Act, 42 U.S.C. § 330A–1 (2010).

CHAPTER 1

Anatomy of a Nurse-Led Clinic: An Introduction to the Model of Care

Tine Hansen-Turton, Brian Valdez, Jamie M. Ware, and Eunice S. King

In the past few decades, an innovative model of primary health care has emerged in the form of nurse-managed health centers (NMHCs). With managed care systems and state-level reforms being introduced to try to control health care costs, the nursing profession has had increasing opportunities to demonstrate the ability to contribute in the areas of health care access, quality, and cost-effectiveness (Lang, 1996). In a landmark randomized control study, Mundinger and colleagues (2000) found that outcome measures such as satisfaction ratings, health service utilization rates, and health status were comparable between advanced practice nurses (APNs), or nurse practitioners (NPs), and physicians. Such studies affirm that NPs can play a vital role in health services in today's environment.

While NMHCs play a key role in improving the quality of life for many people, they face a number of challenges. Because they are innovative models, they often find obtaining necessary mainstream funding to be problematic. Some centers have had to close due to a lack of funding, even though they have been shown to have a positive impact on the health care delivery system. Other obstacles to sustainability include legal, regulatory, and research issues.

BACKGROUND: ORIGINS OF THE NMHC MODEL OF CARE

While today's health centers trace their immediate roots to changes in national health care laws that began in the mid-1960s, the nursing model of holistic care that integrates health promotion with primary care and focuses on serving vulnerable populations dates back to the late 19th century. As far back as the 1890s, visionaries such as Lillian Wald and Margaret Sanger founded the Henry Street Settlement to provide health care to the poor in New York City and opened the first birth control clinic, respectively. These were the earliest nursing service models, and both women were pioneers in the public health movement. Almost three decades later, in the 1920s, Mary Breckinridge, a certified nurse–midwife who had graduated from St. Luke's Hospital School of Nursing in New York, studied public health nursing at Columbia Teacher's College, and completed her education in Great Britain to become a certified nurse–midwife; she became concerned about the lack of accessible health care for childbearing women and young children, except for an occasional physician and untrained "granny midwives," in mountain-ous eastern Kentucky. Seeking to improve the status of maternal–child health in the region, Ms. Breckinridge established the Kentucky Committee for Mothers and Babies, a forerunner of the Frontier Nursing Service (Bartlett, 2008, pp. 39–74). By 1930, the Frontier Nursing Service comprised six very small centers, each managed by an educated nurse or nurse–midwife, and each provided midwifery, sick care, routine immunizations, and checkups for infants and preschoolers within a five-mile radius. Most of the care was delivered in homes by nurses on horseback. The centers were financed in part by a $1 annual prospective payment, in either cash or goods, from every household (Glass, 1989). Challenges faced by those centers were similar to those faced by today's NMHCs: funding, recognition of nurses' importance as providers of care to underserved populations, and scope of practice issues.

When the Social Security Act of 1935 was passed and it appropriated money (a) for nurses to work with state and local health departments to estab-lish health organizations to monitor and protect the health of the community and (b) to train public health nurses (PHNs), public health nursing depart-ments or divisions were established within many municipal or county depart-ments of public health. Although the PHNs provided some care to the sick in their homes, their focus was largely on preventive services, such as administer-ing immunizations, performing well-child checkups, conducting screening for communicable diseases, and tracking the contacts of patients with communi-cable diseases such as tuberculosis or venereal diseases. While PHNs always functioned very autonomously, they worked collaboratively with physicians, who conducted physical assessments, diagnosed, and prescribed treatments (Health Resources and Services Administration, Bureau of Health Professionals, Division of Nursing, 1997 [see "The Role of the Division of Nursing in the Development of NMHCs"]). It was not until the mid-1960s, when educational programs were developed to prepare nurses for expanded roles and legislation was passed that allowed nonphysicians to provide primary care, that nurses were able to become primary care providers (PCPs) and could thus develop the model of nurse-managed health care as it emerged in the late 1970s and 1980s.

THE ROLE OF THE DIVISION OF NURSING IN THE DEVELOPMENT OF NMHCs

The Division of Nursing (DoN)—an organizational unit within the Bureau of Health Professions, one of the four divisions within the Health Resources and Services Administration (HRSA) of the U.S. Department of Health and Human Services (DHHS)—has played a very important role in the emergence of the NMHC model of health care delivery. Historically, the DoN has been the federal agency responsible for providing the national perspective on the nursing workforce, nursing practice, and nursing education. Its contributions to the NMHC movement have included (a) support for the creation of the NP role and (b) advocacy for federal funding to support the development of models of health care for the underserved, one of which was the NMHC.

In 1965, the Commonwealth Foundation supported an innovative project designed by Loretta Ford, RN, and Henry Silver, MD, at the University of Colorado to prepare PHNs to provide comprehensive, well-child primary care in ambulatory settings. An evaluation funded by the DoN documented the NPs' competence and found that 75% of well and ill children in ambulatory settings could be independently managed by pediatric NPs.

In 1968, the DoN, under its project grants, began to fund innovative patient care and educational programs that prepared nurses to practice in expanded roles, such as NPs. In 1971, the report *Extending the Scope of Nursing Practice* concluded that in order for the nation to provide equal access to health care for all its citizens, the practice of nursing should be expanded to include many responsibilities that were traditionally performed only by physicians. Consequently, the Nurse Training Act of 1971 broadened Title VIII authority and earmarked funds to encourage advanced nursing roles (e.g., NPs, clinical specialists, and nurse-midwives) and to increase resources for underserved areas (HRSA, 1997).

By the late 1970s, with the advent of NP programs, schools of nursing were emphasizing the importance of faculty clinical practice in order to maintain and demonstrate expert clinical competence. Some schools, such as the University of Massachusetts Lowell, established NP faculty-run clinics that simultaneously provided a site for faculty to practice and a clinical practice site for NP students. Through Section 3 of the Nurse Education Amendments of 1985, which extended Title VII of the Public Health Service Act, the DoN's Special Projects Program was authorized to fund projects that improved access to nursing services in noninstitutional settings (Clear, Starbecker, & Kelly, 1999). It was under this initiative that funding was available to support NMHCs established by schools or departments of nursing. Support for these centers increased dramatically over the next several years from 2 centers receiving support in 1986 to 9 in 1987, 13 in 1988, 15 in 1990, and 17 in 1992 (Starbecker, 2000). Requirements for receiving funding under this program were the following:

- The academic-based nurse-managed center operated under the administrative aegis of the school of nursing that operated it.
- The center was staffed by faculty and students in the affiliated school of nursing.
- At least 25% of the students enrolled in the school of nursing obtained clinical primary health care experience in the nursing center.
- The center improved access to primary care in a medically underserved area.
- The center offered programs and services to facilitate the achievement of the Healthy People Objectives for the population served (Starbecker, 2000).

Grants made under this program were 5-year awards and were not designed to be renewed. Five years of funding was considered adequate for a center to become established; to apply for other sources of funding, including credentialing by third-party payers; and to build the practice with sufficient numbers of patients to enable it to become self-sustaining. Initially, this seemed theoretically possible. However, a number of changes within the health care reimbursement milieu prevented the attainment of this goal. First, during the mid-1990s, reimbursement for care to clients enrolled in Medicaid programs shifted from cost-based reimbursement to capitation in response to efforts to rein in health care costs, and this shift resulted in a great reduction in service-generated revenue for the centers. This was particularly problematic for the NMHCs because many of them served a high (30%–50% or greater) percentage of uninsured clients and relied on the cost-based reimbursements to enable cost shifting. Second, insurance regulations in many states prevented the Medicaid insurance companies from credentialing NPs, and even after this changed, many of the centers discovered that the process of applying to become approved Medicaid health maintenance organizations (HMOs) and Medicare providers was very time-consuming, labor-intensive, and fraught with delays of as much as a year. Third, NPs in many states did not have prescriptive privileges, which necessitated greater dependence on collaborating physicians. Finally, there was no reimbursement for health promotion programs, so support for those had to be obtained through grants and contracts with private foundations and public organizations (Hansen-Turton, Ritter, & Valdez, 2009).

WHAT IS AN NMHC?

Following in the footsteps of early nurse-managed centers, the nursing professionals in today's NMHCs provide health care that is responsive to each community's unique needs. Since the late 1970s, in conjunction with the development of educational programs for NPs, faculties in schools of nursing have established NMHCs. In addition to providing necessary services to the community, these linkages have provided clinical sites for educating nurses at all levels and settings for faculty practice. Although academic-based nursing centers are a common model, there are also hospital-based and freestanding community-based NMHCs.

NMHCs are managed and staffed by RNs and APNs, NPs who have advanced education and clinical training in a health care specialty. RNs, NPs, and nurse faculty, as well as clinical specialists and PHNs, generally function as the clinical and executive directors of the health centers. These centers are sometimes known as nursing centers, community nursing centers, or nurse-run clinics. They work in partnership with the communities they serve, often at the invitation of the community, and they are embedded in the core of community life (Hansen-Turton & Kinsey, 2001). Staff includes NPs, RNs, PHNs, mental health therapists, health educators, community outreach workers, collaborating physicians, and other health care professionals. Although some NMHCs are located in the suburbs, most serve vulnerable urban or rural populations who would otherwise not have access to health care services.

The National Nursing Centers Consortium (NNCC) adheres to a modified version of the American Nurses Association's (ANA's) Nursing Centers Task Force definition of nursing centers:

> Organizations that give clients and communities direct access to professional nursing services. Professional nurses in these centers diagnose and treat human responses to actual and potential

health problems, and they promote health and optimal functioning among target populations and communities. The services provided in these centers are holistic, client-centered, and affordable.
Overall accountability and responsibility remain with the nurse
executive/director. Nurse-managed health centers are not limited
to any particular organizational configuration; they can be freestanding businesses or may be affiliated with universities or other
service institutions like home health agencies and hospitals. Their
primary characteristic is their responsiveness to the health needs
of populations. The nurse is responsible for all patient care and
operations. (American Nurses Association, 1987)

While NMHCs share the core elements of the ANA definition, they vary
in their practice models. Services offered at nursing centers range from wellness and health promotion to traditional primary care. Some are for-profit
businesses and others are nonprofit academic centers developed primarily
as student clinical laboratories (Lundeen, 1999), which is reflected in the
mission of these academic-based centers. Nonprofit centers have a mission
based solely on direct service. Centers also vary in reimbursement methods,
which may include any or all of the following: fee for service, sliding fees
(usually based on federal poverty guidelines), grants, third-party payments,
and the cost-based reimbursement available to federally qualified health
centers (FQHCs).

Regarding service delivery, there are two types of NMHCs. Nurse-
managed primary care health centers provide comprehensive primary care,
including integrating health promotion, disease prevention, and disease
management. Nurse-managed wellness centers provide health promotion,
disease prevention, and disease management services in established wellness
centers or through extensive outreach into schools, housing developments,
and community-based agencies. Just like the primary care centers, wellness
centers have partnerships with local community agencies, local governments, and managed care organizations. Wellness centers provide services
to the community that can be grouped into one of four categories: health
teaching, guidance, and counseling (e.g., dental care education, safety education, cardiovascular health, and health and life management); surveillance
(e.g., height and weight measurement, vision and hearing screening, glucose
monitoring, and blood pressure evaluation); providing immunizations; and
administering treatments and procedures (e.g., wound care and first aid).

Today, with burgeoning health care costs and a growing number of
uninsured Americans, access to high-quality, preventive health care is a

key concern for policy makers: NMHCs provide a positive solution to the problem. Along with a tradition of community leadership, NMHCs provide evidence-based care and health care education. NNCC member centers have demonstrated significant positive health outcomes for patients, including decreased emergency room visits, hospital inpatient stays, and use of specialists, as compared with conventional health care providers. Primary care NMHCs report excellent pregnancy outcomes, with some reporting close to 100% normal birth weight infants.

Starting any health care enterprise takes careful consideration and planning. This is particularly true of NMHCs because they are not in the traditional model. It is suggested that the steps outlined in this guide be taken into consideration by any organization that is planning a new health center. Those already in existence can also benefit from the experience put forward here.

REFERENCES

American Nurses Association Task Force to Develop Guidelines for Nurse-Managed Centers. (1987). *The nursing center: Concept and design*. Kansas City, MO: American Nurses' Association.

Bartlett, M. (2008). *The frontier nursing service: America's first rural nurse-midwife service and school*. Jefferson, NC: McFarland & Company.

Clear, J. B., Starbecker, M. M., & Kelly, D. W. (1999). Nursing centers and health promotion: A federal vantage point. *Family and Community Health, 21*(4), 1–14.

Glass, L. K. (1989). The historical origins of nursing centers. In National League for Nursing (Ed.), *Nursing centers: Meeting the demand for quality health care* (pp. 21–34). New York, NY: National League for Nursing.

Hansen-Turton, T., & Kinsey, K. (2001). The quest for self-sustainability: Nurse-managed health centers meeting the policy challenge. *Policy, Politics, & Nursing Practice, 2*(4), 304–309. doi: 10.1177/152715440100200408

Hansen-Turton, T., Ritter, A., & Valdez, B. (2009). Developing alliances: How advanced practice nurses became part of the prescription for Pennsylvania. *Policy, Politics and Nursing Practice, 10*(7), 7–15. doi:10.1177/1527154408330206

Health Resources and Services Administration, Bureau of Health Professions, Division of Nursing. (1997, April). *50 years at the Division of Nursing, United States Public Health Service*. Retrieved from http://www.bhpr.hrsa.gov/nursing/50years.htm

Lang, N. M., Sullivan-Marx, E. M., & Jenkins, M. (1996). Advanced practice nurses and success of organized delivery systems. *The American Journal of Managed Care, 2*(2), 129–135.

Lundeen, S. P. (1999). An alternative paradigm for promoting health in communities: The Lundeen community nursing center model. *Family & Community Health, 21*(4), 15–28. doi: 10.1097/00003727-199901000-00004

Mundinger, M. O., Kane, R. L., Lenz, E. R., Tsai, W., Cleary, P. D., Friedewald, W. T., ...Shelanski, M. L. (2000). Primary care outcomes in patients treated by nurse practitioners or physicians: A randomized control trial. *Journal of the American Medical Association, 283*(1), 59–68. doi:10.1001/jama.283.1.59

Starbecker, M. M. (2000). *Historical perspective of division of nursing legislation* (1956–1998). Paper presented at the Health Resources and Services Administration, Division of Nursing, Nurse-Managed Centers Grantee Meeting, Chevy Chase, MD.

U.S. Department of Health and Human Services Division of Nursing. (2000). *Resource and information guide*. Rockville, MD: Author.

CHAPTER 2

The Independence Foundation's Contributions to the Nurse-Managed Health Center Movement

Eunice S. King

BACKGROUND AND HISTORY OF INTEREST IN NURSING

The Independence Foundation (IF) was founded in 1932 by William Donner to encourage cancer research, following the death of a son in 1929. Over the years, the focus of the foundation's funding changed from cancer and medical research to grant programs in secondary education. In 1960, 6 years following the death of Mr. Donner, the $44 million in foundation assets were split equally to form two new foundations: the Donner Foundation, which moved to New York, and IF, which remained in Philadelphia. Over the next 20 years, IF focused its funding on secondary school endowments, scholarships, and loans, as well as grants to local cultural and arts organizations.

In 1980, concerned about the national nursing shortage and what the foundation could do to attract superior students to the profession, IF's board of directors appropriated $1 million for a pilot program of student aid for nursing education in three Philadelphia-area schools of nursing. Funding for nursing education scholarships continued throughout the 1980s, culminating with a $9 million appropriation to establish IF chairs in nursing in nine national schools of nursing that were affiliated with academic health centers: Case Western Reserve University, Emory University, Johns Hopkins University, New York University, Rush University College of Nursing, Rochester

University, University of Pennsylvania, Vanderbilt University, and Yale University. Cognizant that schools of nursing were historically underendowed, the board hoped that this large appropriation would underscore the importance of nursing education, enable schools to engage in long-term planning, and attract greater numbers of students and faculty to these schools.

THE HISTORY OF IF-FUNDED NURSE-MANAGED HEALTH CENTERS: 1993–2013

In the early 1990s, several administrative changes within IF and its board of directors occurred, sparking a reexamination of the foundation's funding and a discussion about areas of potential funding that could have a positive impact on the lives of people in Philadelphia and the surrounding counties. Of particular interest were programs that provided services to those who did not ordinarily have access to them. This shift in interest, along with the addition of two board members with expertise and knowledge about health care, brought about a shift in funding priorities within nursing that began in 1993. The Honorable Judge Phyllis W. Beck was a member of the Board of Overseers of the University of Pennsylvania School of Nursing and had been introduced to the nurse-managed health center (NMHC) model of care through the school's involvement with one of the newly formed centers in Philadelphia. Susan Sherman was the head of the Department of Nursing at the Community College of Philadelphia (CCP), but she was acquainted with the NMHC's model of care through her work with the National League for Nursing, with which she had been active for many years. Furthermore, as a grant reviewer for the Health Resources and Services Administration's (HRSA) Division of Nursing, the federal agency that awarded grants for academic-based NMHCs, Ms. Sherman had reviewed some of the nursing center grant applications and was acquainted with Dr. Sally Lundeen, the founder of a network of nurse-managed centers in the Midwest. The two had served together on the board of the National League for Nursing and had met when Dr. Lundeen came to the Philadelphia area to speak about nurse-managed centers. Since most nurse-managed centers served the health care needs of underserved populations such as minorities, immigrants, and those with low incomes, directing funding to nurse-managed health care centers and programs enabled the foundation to fulfill its mission of providing services to those without access; was consistent with the movement in nursing education toward health care delivery in the community; and supported nurses' functioning in autonomous roles.

Throughout the next 20 years (1993–2013), the strategies for funding NMHCs changed, in response to societal and health policy changes and to lessons learned from grantees. The initial funding strategy was twofold: (a) to fund a variety of innovative nurse-managed programs that addressed an unmet health care need in the community and (b) to strengthen community health nursing curricula in local schools of nursing through the endowment of chairs and direct grants. From the onset, the IF board recognized that in order to demonstrate the viability of an emerging model of health care, it needed to commit itself to "staying the course" by funding the initiative for many years, which it has done for the past 20 years.

1993–2000: Testing and Refining the Funding Focus for NMHC Funding

To support its commitment to community nursing programs, the IF board committed $3,000,000 to establish four IF chairs in schools of nursing in the Philadelphia area. They were filled by faculty leaders in community health nursing practice and education who supported the development of community-based, nurse-managed health care practices in the Philadelphia region and, over the next several years, worked closely with IF to increase the foundation's understanding of the emerging issues in health care and with NMHCs. Further assistance in guiding the direction of the nurse-managed funding initiative came from an advisory committee comprising members who each brought a different yet complementary perspective to the committee: a nurse who had founded a nurse-managed center; a hospital nurse administrator with expertise in finance and management; and a retired expert in public health nursing.

Prior to the IF's commitment to funding nurse-managed programs and centers, these centers had been in existence throughout the United States, but there had never been a sufficient number in any one geographic location to demonstrate their effectiveness. Many of the existing centers were academic based. While the foundation was interested in funding academic-based programs, particularly ones that provided health services 24 hours a day, 7 days a week, it also wanted to fund NMHCs that were operated by nonprofit, nonacademic organizations so that it could ultimately compare the two models.

As Table 2.1 shows, from 1993 until 1998, IF entertained a wide range of nurse-managed health care proposals. Although the foundation anticipated that some of the funded programs might not survive, it believed that the lessons learned from them would inform an understanding of what made NMHCs viable. Among the programs funded during those first 5 years were an

Table 2.1 Types and Numbers of Nurse–Managed Programs Funded: 1993–2000

Program Type	Number Funded Per Year[1]							
	1993	1994	1995	1996	1997	1998	1999	2000
NMHCs: academic-based, offering primary care plus health promotion	2	2	4	5	6	4	5	5
NMHCs: nonprofit, nonacademic, offering primary care with some health promotion	1	1	1	4	4	5	8	6
Nurse-managed, academic-based health promotion programs targeting underserved population(s)	2	2	2	3	5	1	1	1
Nurse-managed, nonacademic-based health promotion programs targeting underserved population(s)	1	0	1	1	1	3	3	1
Nurse-managed programs offering support & education to cancer patients and their families	1	1	1	1	1	1	1	1
Planning for program development	1	8	1	0	1	1	0	1
Nursing education: scholarships; curriculum changes; minority recruitment	7	0	1	1	0	2	1	1
Infrastructure: programs that support centers broadly (e.g., conferences, software, professional organizations, health policy related)	0	1	1	2	2	3	2	1

[1] Number includes new grants plus prior funding commitments for the year.

interdenominational parish nursing program; a hospital discharge follow-up program for elderly patients; nursing education curriculum enhancements in cultural diversity and community nursing; a women's health promotion center for underserved inner city women; nurse-managed primary care health centers; and a nurse-established center to provide support and education services to cancer patients and their families. In addition to grants to newly established programs, planning grants were made to organizations that were studying the feasibility of establishing a nurse-managed program to address unmet health care needs or that were in the early stages of program development.

Refinement of the Focus

By 1998, changes in the federal and state reimbursement mechanisms for health care, the predominance of managed care organizations (MCOs) within the health care market, and welfare reform, with its far-reaching implications for financial access to health care for the poor, were strong influences on IF's decision to focus its funding on NMHCs that provided primary care in addition to health promotion—that is, wellness and disease prevention programs, family planning, and early childhood intervention assessments. It also recognized the importance of funding projects and organizations that would support the growing number of Philadelphia-area NMHCs that offered primary care.

After the first 5 years of funding under this initiative, it was quite clear that sustaining nurse-managed centers that exclusively provided health promotion services was extremely difficult. In several instances, IF provided the majority of funding; without it, the centers could not and did not survive. In contrast, IF had learned that primary care NMHCs had much greater potential for long-term sustainability. Primary care, behavioral health, and family planning services were all direct health care services that were eligible for reimbursement, albeit at times at a very limited level, whereas the health promotion services were usually not eligible for direct service reimbursement except through grants to support specific programs (e.g., lead poisoning prevention, influenza immunization, smoking cessation). As Table 2.1 shows, by 2000, over half of the grantees were in fact primary care NMHCs.

Infrastructure

Changes in health care reimbursement regulations during this period underscored the need to educate health policy makers, at all levels, about nurse practitioners (NPs) and NMHCs, so that the centers could receive reimbursement and also demonstrate their value in meeting the unmet health needs of underserved populations.

Particularly noteworthy during this period were grants that ultimately gave important infrastructure support to the nurse-managed centers that was critical to their subsequent growth and development. In 1997, following a conference to discuss common problems, 13 Philadelphia nurse-managed centers formed the Regional Nursing Centers Consortium (RNCC) to address issues related to reimbursement, to provide national leadership in policy development to overcome obstacles to sustainability, and to educate the public about NMHCs. However, after a year of operating as an all-volunteer organization, it became clear that the scope of work required a full-time paid director and assistant. An IF grant enabled the RNCC to fill these positions.

In the late 1990s and early 2000s, the RNCC successfully worked with the Pennsylvania Alliance of Advanced Practice Nurses to procure the passage of important legislation that laid the groundwork for NPs' being able to practice to the full extent of their licensing and to be reimbursed for their services (Hansen-Turton, Ritter, & Valdez, 2009):

- Act 68 of 1998 provided a legislative definition of primary care providers (PCPs) that specifically included NPs and enabled NPs to be included on the provider panels of Medicaid MCOs.
- In 2000, legislation granting prescriptive authority for NPs in Pennsylvania was passed.
- SB 1208, passed in December 2002, established the Pennsylvania State Board of Nursing as the sole regulator of NPs and clarified the NP scope of practice.

Another important infrastructure-building project was a series of grants made to facilitate data collection. As early as 1995, IF recognized the importance of the centers' ability to collect data to document their scopes of service and describe the clients served, track health outcomes, and monitor the quality of the health care provided. These data were essential for grant applications and reports and critical for the RNCC's health policy work. During the 1995 through 2000 period, several grants were made to develop and test data collection systems in IF-funded NMHCs.

Thus, by the middle of 2000, IF had accomplished the following:

- It had refined its funding to focus on NMHCs that provided primary health care.
- It had identified the need for and committed funding to an organization that could be the voice of NMHCs (the RNCC).
- Having recognized the importance of data collection by the centers, it funded the development and implementation of data collection systems.

2001 Through 2005: Building Infrastructure and Networks

The years 2000 through 2005 presented financial crises for almost all of the foundation's NMHC grantees, particularly the four academic-based centers. The ending of one-time, nonrenewable grants from HRSA's Division of Nursing combined with limited reimbursement from third-party payers and the large number of uninsured patients being served left the centers with minimal operating revenue. Hence, the general operating support from IF was particularly critical during these years while the centers struggled to become financially viable. The most lucrative strategy for obtaining additional reimbursement (i.e., cost based versus capitation) to offset the cost of providing health care to the large numbers of uninsured clients was to become a federally qualified health center (FQHC) or FQHC look-alike center. (For a comprehensive discussion of this, see Chapters 3 and 4.) However, this was not feasible for the academic-based centers because they could not meet the governance requirement that at least 51% of the board of directors be consumers. Therefore, one strategy the academic centers used was to form affiliations with, or transfer ownership to, existing FQHCs. Although in each instance the exact arrangements differed, each of the four academic-based centers ended up doing this. By the end of 2005, there were two networks of NMHCs in the Philadelphia region. One comprised a formerly academic-based center, an academic-based affiliate, and the two original FQHCs. The other comprised the original FQHC, two formerly academic-based centers, and an affiliate center operated by a nonprofit social service agency. The latter network, the smaller and younger of the two, received funding to hire a part-time network director to assess procedures and operations across the four centers, to create a cooperative working milieu among the clinical directors and staff, and to develop strategies for making the centers' operations more efficient.

During the 2000 through 2005 period, grants for new nurse-managed centers and programs were very limited, largely because of IF's philosophy of staying the course with its existing grantees. Two of the grantees that had received awards during the late 1990s and early 2000s underwent significant administrative changes such that they were no longer nurse managed and did not continue to receive funding. The organization that supported cancer patients and their families had grown and become very successful in cultivating a large base of individual and corporate funders, and by 2005, it no longer received funding from the foundation. In 2001, the foundation did begin funding a children's clinic operated by one of the region's Visiting Nurse Associations (VNAs) and continued its support for the next 10 years to enable the clinic to provide primary care services to uninsured and underserved children.

Two very important programs that received increasing levels of support during this period were the National Nursing Centers Consortium (NNCC) and the purchase of an electronic practice management and health record system for use in the nurse-managed primary care centers. By 2000, the RNCC was making significant headway in educating policy makers about nurse-managed centers and in securing federal technical assistance for centers in the FQHC application process. In 2001, the RNCC's membership, which had grown from 13 Philadelphia-region centers to 36 centers in 10 states, voted to change its name to the National Nursing Centers Consortium. Recognizing the limitations of its then organizational affiliation in fostering future growth, NNCC became an independent 501(c)(3) and forged an affiliation with the Philadelphia Health Management Corporation (a.k.a. Public Health Management Corporation). Rapid expansion within NNCC, in both staff and members, enabled it to focus intensively on educating policy makers and lawmakers about the importance of nurse-managed centers and to procure funding for health promotion programs that provided a source of income for participating centers and garnered national acclaim. However, with growth came the need for increased general operating support and a solid infrastructure. Accordingly, the foundation increased its level of general operating support for NNCC and extended supplemental support throughout this time by providing a deputy director, a junior information technology specialist, a health policy analyst, and health policy consultation.

Essential to NNCC's work in advocating for NMHCs was access to aggregate data about nurse-managed centers and clinical outcomes. IF had recognized this as early as 1995, and during the 1995 through 2000 period, it had made a series of grants to different organizations to develop and implement a data collection system. In 2000, management of this project shifted entirely to NNCC and to IF staff. A grant to NNCC in 2000 provided salary support for a part-time information technology consultant who oversaw implementation of the access program in the four pilot centers and created a central NNCC database. However, by the time the system was built and installed in all of the centers, it had been found to lack flexibility in many areas, particularly reporting, and was very limited in the kinds of data that could be collected. As the centers grew, it was clear that an electronic practice management system could facilitate the centers' efficient management of all aspects of their business operations and the electronic health record (EHR) would enable them to more effectively document the care provided to patients, track client health outcomes, and document the quality of care. Accordingly, in 2001, at least 2 years prior to the announcement of the utilization of EHRs as a federal priority, the IF board appropriated $500,000 for the purchase of an electronic practice management and health record system to be implemented in seven of its Philadelphia grantee centers.

Another important project designed to provide data for NNCC about the scope of services and clients served through the nursing centers' health promotion programs was directed by CCP's Department of Nursing, with funding from the foundation. Building on its work in the 19130 Zip Code Project (which CCP promoted as a "wellness center without walls"; see Chapter 14), and recognizing the importance of collecting data that documented its activities, CCP embarked on a rigorous project to develop and test an instrument for collecting health promotion data. From 2000 through 2004, IF funded the development and testing of a data collection tool (see The Zip Code Project Data Collection Tool: An Example of Undergraduate Postclinical Documentation section in Chapter 13) by CCP and four other nurse-managed centers. This tool was often utilized by nursing students as part of their clinical practice to describe the demographic characteristics of their clients, the scope of services provided, and the number of program participants. CCP's IF internship program, initiated in 1996, was an integral part of this project—the interns worked closely with faculty and students in using the data collection tool. Although the intern program had to be phased out in 2009 due to the withdrawal of its primary funding partner, this project continued to receive funding and to be utilized by several nurse-managed, primarily academic-based health promotion centers for the next 10 or more years. The tool underwent several revisions to improve user access and increase the level of specificity of data about the designated programs offered through the centers.

From 2000 to 2005 and beyond, the foundation continued its policy of providing technical assistance, consultation, and support for its grantees. The program officer for the nurse-managed initiative, in addition to managing the implementation of the software system, assisted NNCC in reviewing and editing grants and reports, convened monthly data committee meetings, and met with grantees, at their request, to give advice and guidance around a number of issues. In addition, grantees were invited to attend workshops conducted by Sue Heckrotte, another IF program officer, on topics such as board development and fund-raising. A third kind of assistance was the foundation's facilitation of connections between NNCC and area NMHCs and health policy officials and potential funders. For example, in October 2003, IF hosted a luncheon for Philadelphia-area funders, members of Delaware Valley Grantmakers, to learn more about NNCC and NMHCs through a brief presentation and site visit. During this meeting, IF and NNCC met the vice president of social mission programs from Independence Blue Cross, which subsequently awarded grants to NNCC as well as to several of its Philadelphia-region member NMHCs. The period 2000 through 2005 was a time of great change in organizational affiliation for the centers. IF funding was crucial for enabling many of the centers to continue operation while they explored and implemented strategies that would bring them greater financial security. In addition, recognizing the problems inherent in an organization's dependence on a limited funding stream, IF endeavored, successfully, to bring the attention of other foundations to the NMHC movement.

Challenges Identified From the First 10 Years of Funding

In May 2005, Dr. Eunice King, the program officer for the initiative, completed an analysis of the first 10 years of funding NMHCs. The data that informed the analysis came from several sources:

- In-depth reports on each of the 10 NMHCs that were grantees during and immediately prior to 2000 to 2004. Each report was verified and corrected based on interviews with center directors and staff, with the final drafts being sent to each director for final approval.
- Observations of each of the centers between 2000 and 2004.
- A group discussion held with the directors of 8 of the 10 centers.
- An interview with the NNCC executive director.

The biggest challenge facing the majority of the NMHCs during the period of study was achieving financial sustainability without compromising the centers' mission of providing holistic, comprehensive health care to underserved, indigent populations. Achieving financial sustainability depended on careful business planning, maximizing revenue, and operating as productively and efficiently as possible (King, 2008).

Lessons Learned From the First 10 Years of Funding

- *NMHCs have a difficult time surviving within an academic environment.* By the end of 2005, only one of the original four academic-based centers in Philadelphia was still managed at least in part by the university. The difficulties experienced by these centers may be attributed to the organizational structure, which prevents the centers from obtaining FQHC status—the only way of obtaining cost-based reimbursement in the Philadelphia area—and, in some instances, to the lack of fit with the university's mission and priorities. Furthermore, the academic administrative and fiscal

systems sometimes compromised a center's ability to operate as efficiently as it might have within other organizations. However, in academic
institutions where the nursing center helps fulfill the institution's mission
and priorities, the support the institution can provide may strengthen the
center and broaden the range of health care programs that can be provided to its clientele. The Philadelphia experience vis-à-vis academic-
based nursing centers was consistent with nationwide trends. A survey
of academic-based NMHCs conducted by the University of Michigan in
2003–2004 found that 22 out of the sample of 161 had closed within the
preceding 5 years (Sebastian, 2004). Seventy-seven percent of those cited
financial reasons as the primary reason for closing, with the remainder
citing staffing problems or shifting priorities within the school itself. Similarly, another study of the decline in academic-based NMHCs conducted
by Campbell (2003) also found the primary reason for their decline to be
insufficient revenue, primarily due to loss of patient base and inadequate
reimbursement from managed care contracts. An analysis of six NMHCs
affiliated with the University of Michigan (Pohl, Vonderheid, Barkauskas,
& Nagelkerk, 2004) found that in all but one of the centers, the percentage
of overall budget being subsidized by the university was roughly equivalent to that provided through supplemental grants awarded to FQHCs.
It is therefore not surprising that so many of the academic-based centers
were forced to close; few academic institutions are able to provide that
level of subsidy.

- *Survival of the nurse-managed center model of care depends very much on health
  policy issues related to practitioner reimbursement and credentialing and on
  health policies that favor their survival.*
- *The development or availability of business expertise is essential to the successful
  and efficient operation of the nurse-managed centers.*
- *Recruitment and retention of staff with the right combination of clinical skills, a public
  health/community perspective, sensitivity to the community, and a fit with existing
  staff are essential to maintaining community support and to a center's productivity.*
- *A collaborative, cooperative relationship with the community being served is essential.* The most effective way for a center to build this relationship is through
  a highly engaged community advisory board, which can provide the center
  with feedback about its reputation in the community, community needs,
  and connections to important community stakeholders and programs.
  Most centers' clients are referred through word of mouth, thus making the
  community's perception of a center and its reputation extremely important. (Chapters 9 and 10 vividly describe the importance of this.)

2006–2013: Using the Lessons Learned to Support Service Expansion and Strengthen Infrastructure

By 2006, communities' acceptance and support for the nurse-managed centers had been obtained, many centers had grown such that they had a professional business infrastructure, and staff were becoming more sophisticated about how to operate NMHCs as businesses. However, the work of educating government officials about nursing centers and of effecting favorable policies related to ongoing financial support, reimbursement, and NPs' functional autonomy remained. As a "new" model of health care, NMHCs were only going to be able to survive based on their ability to weather current and future health care crises. They had to be prepared for possible health care system changes before they were implemented, and they needed to ensure that their interests would be represented. Finally, the newly formed networks of NMHCs were experiencing a time of tremendous growth and challenges. In many instances, grants associated with new FQHC service points had brought additional funding that enabled the centers to expand their service capacity, but integrating new centers and staff into existing ones to create networks brought many challenges. To best support the centers, IF used the following tenets to guide its grant making during the 2006 to 2014 period:

- *NNCC's work was seen as critical to providing a strong external infrastructure for the centers and in some cases to supporting the centers' internal infrastructures.* Increasing the visibility of nurse-managed centers, cultivating relationships with influential government officials, monitoring forthcoming changes in the health care delivery system, mobilizing centers nationwide, and implementing strategies to strengthen the position of NMHCs as mainstream health care providers would continue to be very important and were at the heart of NNCC's mission. IF recognized that ongoing support for the nurse-managed model of care from within the nursing profession had to be garnered and knew that NNCC had already formed collaborations with many national nursing organizations. Also of high importance was NNCC's consultation services to financially struggling NMHCs and the health promotion program grants it secured on behalf of participating centers.
- *Nurse-managed centers must document that they deliver high-quality health care that leads to improved health outcomes.* Implementing the EHR software purchased by IF for use by eight of the Philadelphia centers provided the data collection infrastructure required for this documentation. NNCC's process evaluation study, which was funded by the Centers for Medicare and

Medicaid (CMS), demonstrated that care provided by NMHCs resulted in health outcomes that were equivalent to or better than those achieved by providers in comparable community health centers that served a similar population of clients (Hansen-Turton, Line, O'Connell, Rothman, & Lauby, 2004). This study was the first attempt to look at quality from the perspective of provider practices and health outcomes. Prior to this study, quality of care in the nursing centers was assessed solely by patient satisfaction surveys, which measure only patients' opinions about how care is delivered. However, during the study's data analysis, a number of problems were identified that related specifically to provider interpretations of diagnostic and procedure codes, and measures had to be taken to ensure accuracy and consistency in coding across providers prior to the setup and implementation of the electronic medical record system.

- *The NMHC grantees were at different stages in their development, often facing unique challenges and funding needs. Therefore, general operating grants for the centers would allow them the most flexibility to use the funding most effectively.*

At the beginning of 2006, IF was funding eight nurse-managed primary care centers—including one with three locations—two nurse-managed health promotion centers that provided nursing services to individual clients; one academic-based health promotion center that provided a variety of group health promotion activities to schools, day care centers, and senior centers, along with a few health promotion and educational sessions with individuals; and a VNA that provided intensive case management and NP services to chronically ill, often homebound, clients. Of the eight primary care NMHCs, five belonged to one of the two NMHC networks, and by 2006 or shortly thereafter, all five had become FQHCs. The remaining three were part of other nonprofit organizations:

- One health center was part of a social service organization that provided social and educational services to the Mexican immigrant population in one of Philadelphia's outlying counties. The health center was granted FQHC status in 2012, but in order to realize the full financial benefits, the center has been challenged to greatly increase its number of Medicaid clients.
- Another health center was part of a suburban Philadelphia hospital system and fulfilled the charitable mission of its parent organization, with 82% of its operating budget provided by the hospital. Sixty-three percent of visits were and continue to be unreimbursed.

- Unique among the non-network centers was a VNA-operated clinic that only served clients from birth through 21 years of age from low-income families and provided health care to residents of an adolescent treatment facility. In 2012, 79% of their client visits were reimbursed through Medicaid, but the reimbursement was less than half of the center's annual budget. It is unlikely that this center would ever be able to become an FQHC, because it is not located in a medically underserved area.

Even after the new FQHCs began to receive the additional reimbursement, funding from IF remained important, even though by this time the percentages of overall budgets contributed by IF grants had decreased considerably. During the economic downturn in 2007, the foundation reduced the size of its grants to the centers, but restricting its funding exclusively to existing NMHC grantees allowed it to continue its ongoing commitment to its core of centers. The only exception was made in 2013 when IF made a grant to a new health center that was started as an FQHC and needed additional funding for marketing and readying a staff to serve the anticipated demand.

During this period, the foundation reinstituted its previous practice of making challenge grants to centers to encourage them to build individual donor bases and cultivate other sources of funding. All of the centers, particularly those that were not FQHCs or that were primarily health promotion centers, were very appreciative of the opportunity to energize their boards for fund-raising and to leverage this funding to obtain additional support. In all instances, the centers successfully met and often exceeded their challenge.

A Period of Major Growth for the Centers

During this period, the centers grew and developed in many ways:

- As Figures 2.1 and 2.2 show, there was a dramatic increase in the number of overall clients served and visits to the centers.
- A major contributor to the centers' growth was successfully building greater capacity to serve more patients and to expand the services offered. Five of the centers moved into new locations that doubled or sometimes tripled their physical capacities, and those moves were associated with rapid growth in the overall numbers of clients served; in some instances, they led to offering additional services such as dental and/or behavioral health. The acquisition of additional space within their existing locations allowed two other centers to expand.

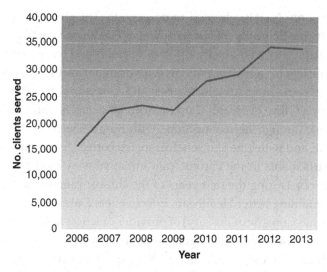

Figure 2.1 Total number of clients served annually by Independence Foundation-
funded NMHCs: 2006–2013.
NMHC, Nurse-managed health center.

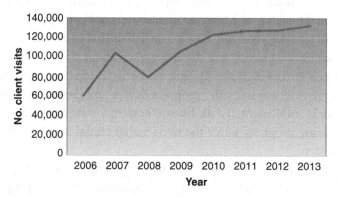

Figure 2.2 Total number of client visits to Independence Foundation-funded
NMHCs: 2006–2013.
NMHC, Nurse-managed health center.

Renovations were often paid for through HRSA grants or grants from
the so-called Stimulus Act of 2009.

- Both NMHC networks were challenged with developing solid infrastructures, integrating the cultures of new centers, hiring and integrating new
  staff, and standardizing clinical practices and office operations across all
  locations.
- Eight of the NMHC grantees were invited to participate in Pennsylvania's Chronic Care Model program that began implementation in 2007 to

2008, the only NMHCs invited to participate. The chronic care program, piloted by the Pennsylvania Department of Health and participating third-party insurers, tracked quality-of-care indicators and participating centers' clinical results in caring for patients with designated chronic illnesses. The invitation came from Ann Torregrossa, JD, Director of the [Pennsylvania] Governor's Office of Health Care Reform, who was familiar with the centers' work through her connections with Susan Sherman, President and CEO of IF, and with Tine Hansen-Turton, Executive Director of NNCC. The other participants in the chronic care initiative were primary care medical practices. During the first years of the chronic care initiative, the focus was on attaining better Healthcare Effectiveness Data and Information Set (HEDIS) measures (see Glossary) of provider practices and health outcomes related to the successful management of adult diabetes (e.g., % of patients with A1c over 9 and/or under 8, LDL under 100, neuropathy screening, annual eye exams, and self-management) and childhood asthma (e.g., use of controller medications), with additional health care measures added each year. As of 2013, all participating centers were tracking and measuring outcomes related to diabetes, hypertension control (BP under 140/90), asthma, and health screenings; assistance with smoking cessation; prenatal care (% of patients receiving care during their first trimesters, % of babies born under 2,500 grams); and depression screening.

- Each center was required to generate periodic reports that were shared with providers to track the progress in meeting the HEDIS goals. Both networks implemented a dashboard system for presenting the data and measuring progress, while the two smaller clinics used a paper reporting system.

- As participants in the chronic care program, all practices including the NMHCs were eligible to receive supplemental funding for their participation and for achieving the provider practice and health outcome goals. However, in order to receive this subsidy, the providers or clinics had to obtain National Committee for Quality Assurance (NCQA) patient-centered medical home (PCMH) recognition, and the amount of reimbursement was dependent on the level of recognition in addition to a number of other factors. (See Glossary for more on the NCQA.)

• By 2009, seven of the eight centers had obtained NCQA Level 1 Medical Home Provider recognition, and the additional center, the children's clinic, had received Level 2 recognition. Throughout the course of their participation in the program, the centers made steady progress in meeting the goals and received additional reimbursement ranging from $15,000 to $175,000 annually. In 2010, these centers were invited to participate in Phase 2 of the Pennsylvania Chronic Care/Medical Home Program. In 2012, six of the centers reapplied for medical home designation and advanced to Level 2. Another center advanced from Level 2 to Level 3 designation. Although the centers continued to receive supplemental payments, during Phase 2, the subsidies were greatly reduced.

- In 2011, the two networks and one additional center began to participate in the CMS Incentive Program to promote the meaningful use of health information technology, which made incentive payments to providers or organizations that could demonstrate their use of EHR capabilities to achieve benchmarks leading to improved patient care. In order to achieve meaningful use, providers had to meet the objectives and measures specified for each successive stage of EHR use. (See Glossary for more on the stages of meaningful EHR use.) The amount of reimbursement a center could receive was based on the number of providers who met the criteria for meaningful use and therefore varied widely. In 2012, the larger of the two networks received a total of $425,000 for 25 providers who met the meaningful use criteria, the other network received close to $179,000 for 15 providers, and the children's clinic received $51,000.

THE NNCC: LAYING THE GROUNDWORK FOR THE GROWTH AND RECOGNITION OF NMHCs

Much of NMHCs' growth and increasing recognition during this period would not have been possible without the work of the NNCC. The importance of this organization to the centers' growth and long-term sustainability was abundantly clear to IF and was the reason for IF's constant support for the organization. Throughout this time period, NNCC's work was guided by its overarching goals of providing national leadership in identifying, tracking, and advising on health care policy; positioning NMHCs as a recognized, cost-effective, mainstream model of health care delivery; and fostering partnerships with people and groups with similar goals. Its activities and strategies were focused on the Philadelphia region and Pennsylvania as well as nationally. Very important during this period were its efforts, along with those of IF, to ensure that NMHCs and advanced practice nurses (APNs) were included in the "Prescription for Pennsylvania," Governor Rendell's plan for health care reform. NNCC worked with the director of the Governor's Office of Health Care Reform and others to ensure that APNs' ability to provide primary care would be expanded and that NMHCs would be included in the Chronic Care Initiative, a program of the Pennsylvania Chronic Care Management, Reimbursement, and Cost Reduction Commission. A total of 400 PCPs, including both of the Philadelphia-area NMHC networks' centers and two other non-network centers, participated. By this time, all but one of the participating nurse-managed centers were fully operational with their EHRs, funded initially by IF, which greatly facilitated the generation of the monthly reports that tracked their progress in meeting the health outcome and provider practice goals. Participation in this initiative brought formal recognition among national policy makers of their ability to produce health outcomes equal to those of other PCPs and additional revenue for results achieved, and, most importantly, it positioned them for participation in future, similar programs.

Each center's level of additional reimbursement was determined by its level of NCQA PCMH home recognition. Initially, NCQA did not confer recognition on NMHCs, but largely through the efforts of NNCC and other groups, it changed its policy in 2010 and began to review and grant formal recognition to NMHCs. As noted previously, by the end of 2013, six of the centers had achieved Level 2 recognition and one had reached Level 3.

With the passage of the Affordable Care Act (ACA) in 2010, NNCC faced many opportunities and challenges to its goal of establishing NMHC as a mainstream model of health care, demanding an increased focus on its national activities. The ACA recognized NMHCs as health care entities through its authorization of $50 million for an NMHC program to be run by HRSA and another $15 million for NMHCs through the Comprehensive Primary Care program. Largely due to the political and economic climate, this money was never appropriated, although NNCC has been successful in obtaining NMHC funding through other appropriations. For example, the Senate Labor, Health, and Human Services subcommittee has given an "expectation" of $5 million for NMHCs in fiscal year (FY) 2014.

Missing from the ACA regulations for health insurers listed in the health insurance exchanges is the specific inclusion of NMHCs in the definition of essential health providers; without this, MCOs are not required to contract with these centers. Based on data obtained from national surveys of MCOs conducted by NNCC in 2005, 2007, and 2010, there has been a steady increase in the percentage of MCOs that credential NPs, from 33% in 2005 to 53% in 2007 and 75% in 2010. Nonetheless, there remain 25% that do not.

Largely due to NNCC's efforts and its collaborating organizations, the Institute of Medicine's report on the future of nursing, released in 2011, emphasizes the importance of nurses' ability to function to the full extent of their education and training. The many activities undertaken by NNCC to bring attention to NMHCs include preparing legislative briefings for delegates of senators and representatives, writing policy briefings and materials, participating on national health care-related committees, cultivating relationships with policy makers, and maintaining strong relationships with coalitions that advocate for nurses at the federal level, for example, the Nursing Community, which represents approximately 60 nursing organizations.

To assist centers in planning for long-term sustainability, NNCC has maintained an active program of providing technical assistance. In addition to convening members once a year for a conference, NNCC provides workshops, training sessions, and webinars on a wide array of relevant topics. It also assists centers that are considering applying or preparing applications to become FQHCs, with the most recent successes being the awarding of FQHC status to two Philadelphia-area centers. A health center empowerment grant has enabled NNCC to provide technical assistance to FQHCs, several of which serve public housing residents.

Finally, one of the ways NNCC has brought both national recognition and sources of additional revenue to the centers is through its many programs to enhance primary care and wellness. Since 1998 to 1999, NNCC has secured grants to reduce lead exposure ("Lead Safe Babies"), improve the management of childhood asthma ("Asthma Safe Kids"), promote smoking cessation, prevent or reduce the impact of heart disease and/or diabetes, and improve the lives of first-time mothers and their children through programs such as the Nurse Family Partnership. All of these programs are grant funded, and most would not be available to the NMHCs as independent applicants because seldom does one individual center have the number of program-eligible clients required by the grant. Approximately 60% to 75% of the grant funding obtained by NNCC passes through to the centers to implement these programs.

A growing focus of NNCC activities is applied research, specifically research that identifies health care-related needs such as the data obtained from the periodic surveys of MCOs regarding their credentialing of NPs and demonstrating the effectiveness or ineffectiveness of health programs. For the past 10 years, NNCC has recognized the importance of having a network of collaborating centers that would participate in health care outcome-related research. It has formed such a network of centers in the Philadelphia region—most of whom have been IF grantees—the Keystone Community Health Alliance. Recently (as of this writing in 2014), NNCC received HRSA expansion funding to enhance its technical infrastructure.

Although NNCC has made much progress in positioning NMHCs as a recognized, cost-effective mainstream model of care, much work remains, and the activities to be undertaken are constantly emerging in response to the ever-changing landscape of our current health care environment.

GLOSSARY

Meaningful Use

"Meaningful use" of health information technology refers to the standards developed by the CMS's incentive programs that hospitals and providers must meet to demonstrate that they are using the capabilities of EHRs to achieve benchmarks that lead to improved patient care. The incentive program was developed to encourage widespread EHR adoption and use among providers.

- **Meaningful use standards align closely with the NCQA PCMH;** that is, they provide patients with summaries of each clinical visit, reconcile medication lists, record patient health practices, and report HEDIS quality measures.
- **EHRs** are widely recognized for their importance in providing health practitioners with prompts to perform specific procedures, for example, measure weight, refer for screening tests, and track patients' responses to health care.
- In order to achieve meaningful use, **providers must meet the objectives and measures specified for each successive stage of EHR use**, namely, Stage 1: data capture and sharing; Stage 2: advanced clinical processes; and Stage 3: improved patient health outcomes.
- Once meaningful use has been demonstrated, providers are eligible to receive incentive payments under either Medicare or Medicaid. Because **Medicare does not recognize NPs as providers under this incentive program,** but Medicaid does, the **NMHCs that participate in this program receive payments under Medicaid, which can total as much as $63,750 per provider who demonstrates meaningful use over a 6-year period.**

National Committee for Quality Assurance

NCQA is a private, nonprofit organization that was founded in 1990 to improve the quality of health care in the nation through "measurement, transparency, and accountability" (www.ncqa.org). Formal NCQA recognition is highly regarded as a symbol of an organization's delivery of high-quality health care. NCQA certification or recognition is obtained only after a very rigorous review process, and annual reports on an organization's performance on health care quality indicators are required for ongoing certification. (See the following text for a discussion of HEDIS measures.) At the federal level, NCQA accreditation and its HEDIS performance measures (http://www.ncqa.org/HEDISQualityMeasurement/HEDISMeasures.aspx) were incorporated into many provisions of the ACA, and other policies have built on the work of NCQA, for example, the PCMH.

- Initially, NCQA focused on reporting health plans' performance measurements and published an annual report entitled *The State of Health Care Quality*. More recently, however, **NCQA has developed certification and recognition programs for a broad range of health care providers, including NMHCs,** along with primary care physician practices; case management, accountable care, disease management, managed behavioral health care, and multicultural health care organizations; and health information products, to name a few. The evolving reimbursement milieu of "pay for performance," versus capitation or fee for service, has prompted many of these organizations such as physician practices and NMHCs to seek NCQA recognition.
- **PCMHs,** as conceptualized by NCQA, entail (a) **enhanced access** to care through expanded hours, online communication, and long-term provider–patient relationships; (b) **clinician-led teams of care** providers to address the prevention and management of acute and chronic conditions, and (c) provider–client **shared decision making.**
  - *In order to receive supplemental funding by participating in the chronic care program, providers must have NCQA PCMH recognition, and the amount of reimbursement depends on the level of recognition in addition to other factors.*
- Since its inception, NCQA has convened large employers, policy makers, physicians, patients, and health plans to build consensus around important health care quality issues, for example, identifying and measuring health care quality indicators and identifying strategies for promoting health. The **NCQA formula for health care quality improvement is to measure, analyze, and improve.**
- In order to measure health care quality, NCQA developed **a set of health care performance indicators that has become the gold standard for measuring health care quality, HEDIS,** which was launched in the mid-1990s and is used by more than 90% of the nation's health plans, health care providers, employers, and regulators.

• **HEDIS includes** a set of **technical specifications for how indicators are to be measured and reported,** thus ensuring the standardization of measurement and reporting that is essential for making valid comparisons across providers, organizations, and/or health plans. HEDIS measures are **continuously updated** through input from a number of different advisors, constituents, and experts **to ensure** that they are (a) **important issues** to be addressed, (b) **scientifically sound**, and (c) **feasible** to implement.

HEDIS currently comprises a set of more than 60 standards in more than 40 areas of health care. Examples of health care issues for which HEDIS measures have been developed include smoking cessation, antidepressant medication management, breast and cervical cancer screening, immunizations, diabetes care, hypertension control, and prenatal and postpartum care, among others.

REFERENCES

Campbell, L. (2003). Out of the briar patch: Diffusion and sustainability of nurse-managed practice. *Dissertation Abstracts International.* (UMI No. 3086272)

Hansen-Turton, T., Line, L., O'Connell, M., Rothman, N., & Lauby, J. (2004). The nursing center model of health care for the underserved. Submitted to the Health Care Financing Administration in fulfillment of HCFA (Contract No. 18- P91720/3-01). (Available from Tine Hansen-Turton, Executive Director, National Nursing Centers Consortium, Centre Square East, 1500 Market Street, Philadelphia, PA 19102.)

Hansen-Turton, T., Ritter, A., & Valdez, B. (2009). Developing alliances: How advanced practice nurses became part of the prescription for Pennsylvania. *Policy, Politics and Nursing Practice, 10*(7), 7–15. doi:10.1177/1527154408330206

King, E. (2008). A 10-year review of four academic nurse-managed centers: Challenges and survival strategies. *Journal of Professional Nursing, 24*(1), 14–20. doi:10.1016/j.profnurs.2007.04.003

Pohl, J., Vonderheid, S., Barkauskas, V., & Nagelkerk, J. (2004). The safety net: Academic nurse-managed centers' role. *Policy, Politics, & Nursing Practice, 5*(2), 1–11. doi:10.1177/1527154404263892

Sebastian, J. (2004, October). *Organizational and business processes of academic nurse-managed centers: A report from a national survey.* Paper presented at the 2004 Annual Conference of the National Nursing Centers Consortium, Nashville, Tennessee.

CHAPTER 3

Building a Nurse-Managed Clinic

Donna L. Torrisi and Tine Hansen-Turton

HOW TO START A NURSE-MANAGED HEALTH CENTER

The following brief overview is taken from the National Nursing Centers Consortium's (NNCC's) nurse-managed wellness center toolkit (available from www.nncc.us). With the implementation of the Affordable Care Act, there is no doubt that there are renewed opportunities for nurse-managed health centers (NMHCs) to grow and thrive.

An initial determination in planning for an NMHC must be whether the center to be developed will operate as an entity under another corporation, such as a university, hospital, or other nonprofit organization, or if it will be an independent nonprofit 501(c)(3) or a for-profit corporation. There are a number of options available, depending on the auspices under which a health center operates. Most NMHCs today are operated by university schools of nursing and have advisory boards to guide their work. Some health centers have the opportunity to obtain federally qualified health center (FQHC) status under the U.S. Department of Health and Human Services (DHHS) Health Resources and Services Administration (HRSA), which affords the opportunity for higher reimbursements and federal malpractice insurance. This determination regarding status should be made as quickly as possible. Assistance can be obtained from HRSA staff or the NNCC, which might connect the new center with an experienced nearby community health center or FQHC. New center managers might want to visit both FQHCs and other types of providers to gain information and explore potential affiliations or partnerships. Assistance may also come from university deans or lawyers or potential partners such as area hospitals. Filing for nonprofit 501(c)(3) status should also be initiated as early as possible because this is a long process. Information can be found at the Internal Revenue Service (IRS) website, www.irs.gov/charities/index.html.

Governing or Advisory Board

A board must be created early in the process of developing the health center because its members will be key to the process. It can be an advisory board for a center that will operate under another organization, or a governing board for independent organizations. Board members may be potential health center users (51% are required for FQHC boards), representatives of health center partners, or experts regarding legal issues, quality of care, or fund-raising. A board should comprise dedicated people who are committed to the health center's mission and willing to work with the management in decision making and problem solving around the development and administration of the organization. Board membership should be such that it represents and is able to serve as a link to the community that the health center serves and reflects the interests and needs of the population. The board should have a diversity of strengths and capabilities to maximize its effectiveness. It must be determined what kinds of skills are needed to start out, and what key community figures might be able to help both in the development process and in identifying potential board members.

A board must be governed through bylaws, which can be developed using those of another organization as a model and which should be reviewed regularly. (Appendix B presents an example of a health center's bylaws.) A board's most important responsibility is selecting and, where necessary, dismissing the executive director to whom it delegates authority and responsibility for the organization's management and for implementing the health center policy. This responsibility is always part of a governing board's responsibility and sometimes part of that of an advisory board. The roles of the governing or advisory board need to be decided on and spelled out in the bylaws.

Mission

The mission of the organization and of the NMHC should be determined early in the process, understanding that it might be revised over time as the strategic planning process evolves. The mission statement should articulate the center's primary goal(s)—to serve the community, as a faculty practice or learning site for students, and so on—and whether the center will provide primary health care or health promotion services only. The mission and accompanying vision, principles, and/or values will help guide decision making. The mission statement should be short and clear and should convey the center's vision to funders, staff, and patients. For an FQHC, the mission should specifically include the need to provide service to underserved people and to eliminate barriers to access of care.

Licensure, Accreditation, and Status

Licensure

A primary responsibility of the organization is to obtain any required licenses; requirements vary from state to state. In some states, health centers do not need to apply for licensing, though the area where the clinic will be must be zoned for a health care facility. The center director will need to contact the state's health department or the designated regulatory body for requirements. In addition to licensing the facility, the director of the health center must verify that employees are certified or licensed as necessary. Copies of the nurse practitioners' (NPs') current certifications and/or state licenses should be on file at the practice, as should a practice agreement with a collaborating physician specifying what the NPs may do, if this is required by state regulation. Providers must be credentialed with payers to allow the health center to receive payment for services.

Accreditation

Another issue that needs to be considered is whether the organization will seek accreditation. Among the most prominent accrediting bodies for health care entities is The Joint Commission (www.jointcommission.org). This independent group accredits most types of inpatient and outpatient health care facilities, hospitals and health care networks, and health plans. Although accreditation is voluntary, the health care industry and the public view it as a seal of approval for an organization. Specific guidelines for accreditation can be accessed via the Internet.

FQHCs that do not obtain The Joint Commission accreditation are approved through a federal Primary Care Effectiveness Review (PCER). This extensive evaluation, conducted by the U.S. Bureau of Primary Health Care (http://bphc.hrsa.gov), consists of an in-depth assessment of primary care services, policies and procedures, governance, and fiscal operations carried out by a team of experts over the course of several days. The team provides a written assessment, and the health center must develop a correction plan in response to any issues cited; there will be a timeline for the plan's completion. The PCER process is repeated every 5 years.

Determination of Status

There are a number of status options available to NMHCs. They can provide full primary care services or focus on health promotion, disease prevention, and education and wellness. Those primary care models that are serving underserved areas and/or populations can also seek FQHC status, but the requirements are stringent and difficult for some centers to meet. The advantages of FQHC status are that FQHCs are eligible to receive cost-based rates for Medicaid and Medicare services and, if they receive a federal health center grant, they are eligible for federal malpractice coverage, saving them a great deal of money every year. The reimbursement rates are calculated based on the cost of services provided in the first 1 or 2 years the center is in operation. The rates are then trended upward based on inflation and are otherwise difficult to change, unless new services are offered. Federal malpractice insurance is available to the FQHC's direct employees and contractors, but not to those who are contracted through a practice.

Some health centers will not qualify for FQHC status. The most common type of center, the academically based model, which makes up 60% of the members of the NNCC, generally does not qualify. Most of these centers are founded by schools of nursing and are operated by the schools as faculty practices and venues for student learning. Because they are under the auspices of the schools with which they are affiliated and their directors and staff are employed by the schools, these centers have advisory rather than governing boards. These advisory boards generally do not meet FQHC governance requirements, namely, that a minimum of 51% of an organization's governing board members must be health center users and that the board should control health center policy and services and have the authority to hire and dismiss the director. The same problem is often found with hospitals and other multiservice corporations that develop health centers. The level of independence and control vested in the board is key to FQHC status.

There are some ways that such organizations may be able to become eligible to be FQHCs. In some cases, HRSA waivers that allow health centers operated by other entities to be governed by separate advisory boards that have adequate levels of control can be obtained when special populations, such as public housing residents, the homeless, or migrant workers, are to be served. Public entities, such as public universities, that meet the FQHC standards other than those regarding governance can apply for FQHC look-alike status, which allows them to obtain cost-based reimbursement but not malpractice insurance. Look-alike centers can compete for federal grants if they receive a waiver of those requirements. However, a request for such a waiver will likely put the health center at a disadvantage in a highly competitive process, unless (a) the waiver request clearly spells out the authority that will reside with the advisory board and (b) that authority is substantive, as described earlier.

Other ways that academic-based centers can position themselves for FQHC status include spinning off independently governed entities and various types of affiliations with FQHCs. Affiliations need to be very carefully considered, and health centers are advised to discuss the possibilities in detail with HRSA before taking steps in this direction.

Care must be taken to ensure that any affiliations allow the center to meet desired goals and do not conflict with its mission. For instance, affiliation with an FQHC that is not nurse managed may put the nurse-managed status of the health center in jeopardy. Also, only staff employed directly by an FQHC are covered under federal malpractice insurance; employees of a university working under contract are not. If federal funding is requested for an affiliation to give a health center FQHC status, the proposal must be very carefully written to ensure that reviewers are able to ascertain how the affiliation will work and the way governance issues in particular will be addressed.

The legislative definition of an FQHC is as follows:

- An entity that is receiving a grant under Section 329, 330, 340, or 340a of the Public Health Service (PHS) Act
- An entity that is receiving funding from such a grant under a contract with the grantee and that meets the requirements to receive a grant under Section 329, 330, 340, or 340a of the PHS Act
- An entity that, based on HRSA recommendation, the secretary determines meets the requirements for receiving a grant under Section 329, 330, 340, or 340a of the PHS Act
- An entity that is receiving grant funds either directly or indirectly and is defined by the scope of the approved Section 329, 330, 340, or 340a grant application with respect to size, organization structure, and location of the facility or facilities
- An outpatient health program or facility operated by an Indian tribe or tribal organizations under the Indian Self-Determination Act (Public Law 93-638)

- An Urban Indian Health Organization that is receiving funds under Title V of the Indian Health Care Improvement Act for the provision of primary health services
- An entity that was treated by the secretary, for purposes of Part B of Title XVII, as a comprehensive federally funded health center as of January 1, 1990

  FQHCs must meet standards in a number of areas:

- Need and Community Impact
  - Demonstrate the need for services in the community based on geographic, economic, and demographic factors; other area resources; and population health status
  - Must serve those most in need within the service area, including low-income individuals, the uninsured, minorities, pregnant women, the elderly, migrant or seasonal farmworkers, and, where appropriate, those with special needs
  - Must serve a designated Medically Underserved Area (MUA) or Medically Underserved Population
- Health Services
  - Applicant must provide the following, either directly, through contract, or through formal referral arrangements with accountability to the applicant: primary health care services by physicians, NPs, and physician assistants (PAs); diagnostic laboratory services and x-ray services; case management; pharmacy services needed to complete treatment; mental health services; prenatal care; preventive dental services; emergency services; and transportation for patients who would otherwise lack access.
  - All contracted services must remain under the governance, administration, clinical management, and quality assurance (including record review) of the applicant organization. This will be affirmed through a description of accountability for all contracted services and the submission and review of contract documents for any contracted services comprising more than 10% of costs submitted by the entity for payment.
  - The applicant must ensure full representation of the target population in providing FQHC services (i.e., the population served may not be limited by age or gender). This requirement may be achieved through the prime contractor or a network arrangement that meets the contracting requirements described earlier.
  - Applicant must demonstrate that it maintains a core staff of full-time primary care providers (e.g., physicians and NPs, PAs, certified nurse–midwives).

- Applicant must demonstrate that there is a sufficient but not excessive number of primary care providers in relation to the persons served.
- All primary care providers, with the exception of certain National Health Service Corps providers, are licensed to practice in the state where the center is located.
- Applicant's primary care providers have hospital admitting privileges or, in cases in which this is not feasible, the applicant has referral arrangements in place for hospitalization and discharge planning, which ensures continuity of care.
- Services must be available to all, regardless of ability to pay.
- The applicant must use a charge schedule with a corresponding discount schedule based on income.
- The applicant must be open at least 32 hours per week, providing services at times that meet the needs of the majority of potential users. Applicant should indicate whether early morning, evening, or weekend hours are scheduled each week.
- The applicant must provide professional coverage during hours when the center is closed, demonstrating firm arrangements for after-hours coverage by their own providers and, if necessary, other community providers. This system must ensure telephone access to a provider who is part of the center's after-hours system.
- The applicant must have an ongoing quality improvement (QI) program that identifies problems and allows for necessary actions to remedy problems.
- Management and Finance
  - The applicant's organization should have a line of authority from the board to a chief executive (president, CEO, or executive director) who delegates, as appropriate, to other management and professional staff, including a finance director and a clinical and/or medical director. An organization chart reflecting these positions and their relationships should be maintained and periodically updated by the chief executive and provided to the board.
  - The applicant must have systems that accurately collect and organize data for reporting and that support management decision making. The applicant must be able to integrate clinical, utilization, and financial information to reflect the operations and status of the organization as a whole.
  - The applicant must have accounting and internal control systems that are appropriate to the size and complexity of the organization.

- The applicant must have in place written billing, credit, and collection policies and procedures, including a system for billing patients and third parties within 45 days of a service's being rendered; a procedure for aging accounts receivables, producing appropriate aging reports, and following up on overdue accounts to ensure collection; and a procedure for handling bad debts on a regular basis.
- The applicant must demonstrate that an annual independent financial audit is performed in accordance with federal audit requirements.
- If problems are cited in the audit or report on internal controls, these problems must be explained, and adequate procedures must be in place to correct them.
- The applicant must demonstrate that annual revenue equals 90% of expenditures. Revenue and expenditures are to be reported upon application and substantiated by the audit.
- The applicant must demonstrate that it has, or has applied for, a Medicaid provider number as an FQHC.
- The applicant must demonstrate that it is a Medicare provider if it serves patients over 65 or Supplemental Security Income patients.

- Governance
  - The applicant must be a public or private nonprofit entity as certified through federal or state process.
  - The applicant's governing board must have 9 to 25 members, the majority (at least 51%) of whom are active users of the center and who, together, represent the center's user population. The board is expected to meet monthly. When the governing board is a university or other corporation that serves a broader range of constituents, an advisory board that consists of a minimum of 51% health center users may govern the center. In this case, the governing board will not have a majority of health center users, and a waiver may be obtained from the federal government. Waivers from monthly meetings may also be requested. No more than half of the nonuser governing board members may derive 10% or more of their income from the health care industry.
  - If the applicant is a private nonprofit, the governing board must have full authority and responsibility for center operations. Specifically, the board must have the authority to approve the center's budget, approve the selection and dismissal of the top-level management, and set center policies.
  - If the applicant is a public entity, the governing board must have the same authority as that of a private nonprofit organization, except that the public agency may retain the authority to establish general (fiscal

and personnel) policies for the center. There must be a written agreement between the governing board and the public agency, delineating the roles and responsibilities of each entity. The governing board must have the authority to approve the center's budget, approve the selection and dismissal of the top-level management, and set center policies.

- The applicant's bylaws or written corporate policies must include provisions that prohibit conflict of interest or the appearance of conflict of interest by board members, employees, consultants, and those who provide services or furnish goods to the applicant. No board member may be an employee of the center or be an immediate family member of an employee.

FQHC standards are based on sound practice. These standards, other than the specifics regarding governance, were used in developing this guide. Links to FQHC information are available on the NNCC website, www.nncc.us.

Site Selection

Selecting the site for an NMHC requires significant study and planning. It is imperative that the center be located in an area where there is a defined need that is not being met by any other provider(s). This is especially necessary for a center seeking federal funding or FQHC status, since the government, like most funders, does not want to fund duplicate services. Geographic access for the target population, including ease of public transportation and parking, are key considerations. The financial resources available will dictate whether the facility should be rented or purchased. The services to be provided at the health center will determine the size and layout of the physical space.

Zoning is another factor in site selection. Zoning is how the government controls the physical development of land and uses of property; even though a space may have commercial zoning, it is important to know whether or not it can be utilized as a health center. Depending on the local rules and ordinances, some businesses will need a permit or license to operate. An organization would do well to contact local political entities and/or a lawyer early in the process to ensure that sites being considered are viable possibilities.

INITIAL PLANNING

Once a determination has been made as to the type of health center that will be operated and the initial board has been formed, the formal planning for the health center can begin. Sometimes, some of the needs assessment will be done before these determinations are made.

Needs Assessment

Since NMHCs are community focused, a comprehensive, written community needs assessment should be done to ensure that the programs and services that are developed are as responsive as possible to the community. It will be important to identify the population to be served; the community's beliefs, values, and attitudes; and the community's current barriers to accessing quality health care. Assessing the community will provide health care professionals with an understanding of community dynamics and how they contribute to or detract from the population's state of health (Clemen-Stone, 2002). The assessment may also help to identify the population's unmet needs and the health disparities between it and the larger community, as well as avoid duplication of services. This type of needs assessment should be ongoing, because communities are dynamic systems, and continuing changes will affect the need for services (Lundeen, 1999).

The focus of the needs assessment should be on the community's strengths and existing resources. Any community organizations that have similar interests and may be potential collaborators or competitors should be identified and studied. This type of review can reduce the chance of duplication of services and could lead to providing a comprehensive array of services through collaboration, resource sharing, and cost-effectiveness. Other benefits of collaboration or affiliation may be promoting the commitment to community health improvement efforts, activating citizens to participate in health decision making, and promoting a shared vision regarding community health goals and outcomes (Clemen-Stone, 2002).

Local organizations and leaders are invaluable resources because of their links to the community. Utilizing them in developing the center will help to identify gaps in health care services and ensure that the programs developed are suitable to the community's culture. There are several means of assessing communities, including face-to-face interviews with community residents and leaders, town hall meetings, and reviewing community newspapers and organization publications. In addition, organization staff can conduct neighborhood windshield surveys and walking tours, that is, tours of a geographic area at varying times to observe and record information and community characteristics (Clemen-Stone, 2002).

According to Glick and colleagues (1996), the success of a community-based program depends on community member participation and the fostering of a sense of neighborhood "ownership." It is vital that some of the methods noted in the preceding text be used to ensure that, from the outset, the community is aware of the organization's plans; community leaders have real input in the development process; and the services provided by the health center are culturally appropriate and accessible to the target population. Community input should not be limited to the needs assessment and planning process. An organization coming into an underserved community should expect that, initially, community members might be reluctant to trust. This is not surprising, given their history of being used and abused and of broken promises. It is imperative that nursing leaders be sensitive to this and willing to work through difficult issues in order to establish lasting, trusting partnerships. Open dialogue between the organization and the community can help build rapport and trust and is critical to developing culturally appropriate, community-focused services.

Strategic Planning

An organization that is planning to develop an NMHC should first create a comprehensive, written strategic plan that covers 2 to 5 years and includes a long-range financial plan and a capital plan to accomplish determined goals. The strategic plan must have input from the board, staff, and community leaders and should be approved by the board.

An internal assessment should be done that includes a strengths, weaknesses, opportunities, and threats (SWOT) analysis and that considers the organization's resources and staff skills, as well as its limitations. The analysis should consider reimbursement trends and the center's competitive position and should include the following: existing services, services restricted by third-party payers, services expanded to meet third-party requirements, and potential services that provide more comprehensive care (Kinsey & Gerrity, 1997). The board and management should review and either affirm or revise the organization's mission.

The strategic planning effort should use the information from the community assessment, as well as the internal assessment or strategic analysis, to develop a comprehensive plan for services to be provided, collaborations/affiliations to be established, and financial and capital plans that take into account all pertinent issues. The range of services that will be provided both directly and indirectly should be specified. The number of practitioners and support staff needed should be detailed, as should their required credentials. The center's need for volunteers and the ways they can be recruited, used, and monitored should also be considered. The mechanisms for including the community in planning and managing the center and its services should be part of the plan, as should the center's plan for participating in community, local, state, and national networks.

Funding

There are a number of funding options for NMHCs, including federal, state, local, and private grants, state and local contracts, third-party reimbursement, and fee for service (FFS). There are advantages and disadvantages to each option. Because there is not a single model to depend on in establishing a viable financial base, it is important for NMHCs to cultivate multiple funding streams to support the best possible cash flow. Most are supported by a patchwork of public and private funding—financial development requires a great deal of flexibility and creativity.

Federal, State, and Local Grants

Obtaining a major grant can secure a health center's finances for the length of the grant. Such funding can enhance the center's public image and may leverage other funding as well. If an NMHC qualifies as an FQHC, it can receive ongoing funding through the HRSA Community Health Care program. Other time-limited funding includes HRSA Division of Nursing funding.

If it is an option and an NMHC has a significant number of Medicare or Medicaid clients, FQHC status can ensure cost-based reimbursement for Medicaid primary care visits and an augmented rate for Medicare. This can make the difference between a capitation rate of $9.00 per member per month and a per-visit reimbursement rate of $120 per visit, depending on the center's actual cost per visit. HRSA also offers opportunities for FQHCs to obtain funding that allows for service expansions, facility improvements, or special projects focused on reducing health disparities.

The disadvantage of public grants is that they generally come with significant amounts of oversight and regulation and a number of stipulations. Also, grant proposal writing requires a great deal of time and energy, and any resulting award is uncertain.

State and Local Contracts

Contracts with public entities or other organizations may provide reliable and predictable income for the health center as payment for specific services. Again, public contracts usually come with a great deal of oversight and regulation, and contracts with private organizations such as other agencies, businesses, unions, city and state governments, or housing authorities must be constructed carefully to ensure that they are specific about the services that will be covered and those that may be separate from the contract. Contracts cover the ways that disputes are negotiated, and they detail how services are paid for. They are binding, and they must be adhered to even if resources or staffing decline, unless both parties renegotiate the terms.

Family Planning Contracts

It can be worthwhile to have a contract with a local family planning council if one exists in the area. In Pennsylvania, these contracts award annual capitation fees to provider organizations for each patient enrolled in the family planning program. They also bill Medicaid for contracted family planning providers. Fees are a carve-out FFS arrangement from the Medicaid managed care health maintenance organization (HMO). The FFS is in addition to the usual capitation for primary care services.

Fee for Service

The FFS model is a common payment system, one that is adjustable to changing financial conditions. However, health centers must find a balance between setting fees that are adequate to cover the cost of services and the need to avoid overpricing services, which can significantly reduce the center's financial base. The FFS model requires a billing and collection system and, for many centers, the development of a sliding scale fee schedule for patients who are uninsured or underinsured. The sliding scale is usually based on federal poverty guidelines and is required to be based on those guidelines for federally funded programs.

Third-Party Reimbursement

Third-party reimbursement is another common payment system in health care. There are a number of sources of third-party reimbursement. Medicare, Medicaid, insurance companies, HMOs and managed care organizations (MCOs), and businesses that contract for certain services are the major third-party payers. The health center should plan according to the expected mix of payers and rates. The mix will vary, based on the population served, the services provided, and the available sources of payment. One FQHC in Philadelphia strives to maintain a minimum of 60% Medicaid patients, 30% uninsured patients, and 10% patients insured by Medicare or private insurance. One way this is done is to assist patients in establishing their eligibility and applying for Medicaid. Medicare now pays a low fee for each visit, but may soon change to cost-based reimbursement rates similar to those for Medicaid.

Each payer organization has its own reimbursement policies and fee schedules. It is important to designate one person in the organization who will be responsible for having current knowledge about insurer reimbursement processes for third-party reimbursement. Nurse-managed centers will need to obtain a provider number for both Medicare and Medicaid reimbursement. Both of these payers utilize the Health Care Financing Administration (HCFA) Form 1500 for billing. Depending on the insurance company, provider numbers for these may also be required, so it is important to contact each specific company. For MCOs, providers need to request an application for admission as a new provider.

In some parts of Pennsylvania and the nation, HMOs and MCOs are resistant to contracting with independent NPs and NMHCs. Strategic approaches to this issue, spearheaded by the NNCC and nursing leaders, have broken down many of these policies, but they continue to be a barrier in some areas. It is important for a new health center to explore early on in the planning process the carriers that operate in the area, any limitations that exist to third-party reimbursement for nurse-managed services, and any limits on the number of new providers.

The disadvantages of third-party reimbursement are the costly process involved in billing insurers, the sometimes significant delays in payment, the need to track and follow up on denied payments, current procedural terminology (CPT) codes that may limit reimbursable nursing services, and insurance gatekeepers that may limit the number of new providers (Elsberry & Nelson, 1993). Third-party payment is difficult to obtain for health promotion and disease prevention centers, although some centers have received reimbursement for special chronic illness management programs.

Private Philanthropic and Corporate Sources

Finding nontraditional sources of funding, such as private philanthropic foundations and corporations, is important because the pillars of public health—health promotion, health education, and disease prevention—are rarely reimbursed by public sources or patients, even though communities see these as essential, value-added services. However, because a significant amount of time and management energy needs to be devoted to monitoring and applying for such funding and because the success of such efforts is unpredictable, the organization must carefully consider pursuing such funding, and may wish to consider either hiring or contracting for a development director. A good development director can be extremely valuable.

Before seeking private funding, the organization should complete its strategic plan, because many funders require such a plan before considering a grant, particularly for a new organization or program. Case statements should also be developed regarding the specific programs or items for which funding will be requested, including a full discussion of the need for the services, details of the services to be provided and the outcomes to be achieved, and the methods of evaluation to be used. Staff and board members of the organization should consider collecting quotations regarding the program or services from letters, phone calls, testimony at public hearings, or comments in the press. These quotations can then be used on the title page of the grant request, as part of a summary paragraph, in the background section of the request, or when talking about a specific program. Furthermore, these quotations can be used in the annual report or other public relations materials and on the organization's website (Adams, 2002).

In order to identify likely foundation funders, the organization should begin with background research in a directory of foundations (Fazzano, 2002). Starting the search for funders at the local level may be more successful than approaching larger, national foundations. Typically, local foundations tend to fund local organizations. Also, smaller charitable organizations usually have less competition for funds and involve less bureaucracy and oversight (Elsberry & Nelson, 1993). After identifying foundations that share a similar mission, the organization should try to identify people who may know staff or board members of these foundations. A list of organizations the foundations have funded in the past is usually available and informative. In addition, foundations that currently fund or have previously supported the health center may have leads that will help to diversify the organization's funding. If current donors have contacts with other funders, they may be willing to make some introductions.

The personal approach can be helpful in developing relationships with potential funders. For instance, inviting funders to an event is a way to introduce them to the organization's work. Another technique for establishing a relationship is calling funders from time to time for advice or technical assistance, if they are receptive to this. It is important to build credibility with grant makers. Active participation in policy-making activities, advocacy groups, and other organizations can give the health center visibility that will be helpful in the search for support.

Prior to submitting a letter of inquiry, the organization should request the latest application guidelines, an annual report, and other pertinent materials about the funder. The eligibility requirements should be reviewed carefully, and the application guidelines should be followed *meticulously*.

FINANCIAL OPERATIONS

Operating a health center requires financial planning and sound financial management. For this reason, it is important for the health center's strategic plan to include a business plan with at least a 2-year projection of revenue, as well as a capital budget and plan. Funding must be identified and secured and financial management processes in place when operations begin.

Business Planning

A business plan is a management tool. It helps an organization identify financial and other organization goals for the year and monitor achievements and setbacks. Before writing a business plan, it is important to identify the audience who will be using it, other than the organization's management. In particular, business plans often must be submitted to certain funders as part of proposals for funding or progress reports. If an organization's business plan will be sent to potential funders, it must be designed to inform them about the organization as well as the goals and objectives for the year. Components of a business plan might be

- Business description (name, organization background, health center mission, and special features of the services provided)
- Management section (organization structure, roles of key personnel, relevant team experience and capabilities, personnel strategies and issues such as staff recruitment and retention, and service supports such as advisors, boards, and consultants)
- Marketing section (market research studies completed, market niche, competitive analyses)
- Financial section (income statements, balance sheet, cash flow statements, sources and uses of funds, and break-even analysis)
- Critical risks section (internal strengths and weaknesses, external threats and opportunities, competitor strategies, and other possible events that could bring the business to a halt)
- Appendices (purchase orders, contracts, letters of intent, and résumés of management and key personnel)

Financial Management

The NMHC must develop and implement plans to meet its immediate and long-range financial requirements and manage its fiscal affairs. A long-range financial plan and a capital plan should be part of the strategic plan. As noted earlier, the organization must seek revenue that will be adequate to support the services the center is committed to providing, including both government and private sources where possible, seeking diversification and balance for stability. Financial procedures should be developed to ensure that the health center's fiscal affairs are managed according to sound financial principles and in compliance with all laws related to fiscal accountability and governance. Procedures should be written and used to train financial and management staff.

Budget Development and Monitoring

Creating and following a budget are essential to a health center's survival. The annual budget should reflect the center's goals and should be dynamic so that it can be adjusted to reflect changes in the business and economic environment. The budget should consider the funding anticipated during the year, the fixed and incremental operations costs, and any potentially changing costs and conditions. It must also consider the personnel necessary to accomplish long- and short-term goals and staff member workloads. The development of the annual budget should include a review of the long-range financial plan that is part of the strategic plan. The board should approve the annual budget before the beginning of each fiscal year. All significant deviations should be explained, and the board should also approve any resulting changes.

The annual budget includes revenue, operating expenses including state and federal taxes, and cash flow projections. Revenue is the funding that the organization has and plans to acquire to pay the bills. Operating expenses include rent, insurance, payroll costs, taxes, supplies, building maintenance, interests on loans, and overhead. The budget will help forecast the business's cash needs and control expenditures.

The management and board should review fiscal statements no less often than quarterly (monthly for FQHCs) to examine the relationship of the budget to actual expenditures and revenue and to examine issues of fiscal policy, budget preparation, and recommendations by the organization's auditors. Reports to the board should be written and, where possible, copresented by a board member. The board should also receive reports on practices and trends with regard to the agency's contractual relationships.

Financial Accountability

Internal audit functions are carried out regularly throughout the year, including cash reports, bank statement and accounts receivable reconciliations, general ledger account analysis, fee and reimbursement collection, and a comparison of actual expenses with the budget. A full audit should be conducted of the governing organization each year by an independent public accountant selected by the board and should be formally received and accepted by the board. Any recommendations made in the annual audit or by funders should be followed up and reported on to the board.

Financial Procedures

Financial procedures should be designed to provide reasonable assurance regarding the efficiency of center operations, the reliability of financial reporting, and compliance with applicable laws and regulations. Procedures regarding internal controls should include but not be limited to the following:

- Procedures for budget development, monitoring, variance analysis, and audit
- Procedures requiring an accrual method of accounting and prompt and accurate recording of revenue and expenses
- Procedures requiring accurate accounts of units of service provided, timely submission, appropriate follow-up on any denial of coverage or payment, and compliance with applicable regulations, which will provide safeguards against over- or underbilling
- Separation of accounting duties to the extent possible and other methods to prevent and detect fraud or abuse of the controls
- Procedures for preparing any reports required by all funding sources
- Procedures for reviewing and approving payroll expenditures, including time and overtime records and written authorization for new hires, terminations, pay rates, and deductions
- Authorization levels for all other expenditures
- Purchasing procedures, including competitive bidding for major purchases
- Fixed asset procedures and inventory controls
- Review and approval of unplanned expenses and any budget adjustments required by variances

FQHC procedures should also include procedures for completing the Uniform Data Set report and for unit cost assessment. The use of medical group management software should be considered to assist in required cost analysis. Procedures should indicate that all contracts must be reviewed to ensure their compliance with federal requirements and must include language regarding their length and conditions of termination. Contracts for required FQHC services must allow the center to set practice guidelines and review performance.

POLICIES AND PROCEDURES

Policies and procedures guide the work of the health center and promote service quality, consistent performance, safety, sound business practices, and communication of standards and expectations throughout the organization.

They are essential for providing clear guidelines and rationale for staff practice and behaviors. Policies and procedures must be written and should reflect the health center's mission, vision, and goals. Involving staff in developing policies and procedures, whenever practical and appropriate, promotes staff engagement and helps to ensure that procedures are comprehensive and relevant to staff practice.

The board should approve the center's policies. Organization and service procedures are developed by health center management to detail how the policies will be implemented.

Local, State, and Federal Regulations

When developing policies and procedures, the health center should be aware of all local, state, federal, and contractual regulations that impact its operations. State laws govern NMHCs' scopes of practice, prescriptive authority, and collaboration requirements, while state and federal laws address the care of patients covered by Medicaid and Medicare. Governance of NP practice varies by state and may involve oversight by a state board of nursing or joint oversight with a state board of medicine. All states require NPs to hold state licenses as RNs and as certified registered nurse practitioners. Nineteen states require that NPs have master's degrees, and 31 states require that they obtain national certification (Buppert, 1999). NPs' prescriptive authority also varies by state. The *Nurse Practitioner's Business Practice and Legal Guide* is an invaluable resource for state-specific information (Buppert, 1999). Another resource is each state's board of nursing, an appointed board within each state and territory that regulates the practice of nursing. Organizations should stay current on state legislation and be involved in coalitions and task forces that affect the rules and regulations governing nursing practice and NMHCs.

Organization Policies and Procedures

Organization policies outline the broad management and administrative functions of the health center, delineate the broad responsibilities of staff members, establish such basic requirements as the code of ethics and patient rights, and require the maintenance of quality services. These and personnel policies are approved by the board. In addition to fiscal procedures that guide the center's financial operations, organization procedures include those for risk management, personnel, and other administrative areas including guiding the management of information and adherence to the Health Insurance Portability and Accountability Act (HIPAA) requirements; those that establish processes for patient grievances, reporting of incidents and accidents, reportable illnesses and conditions, and child abuse and neglect; and those that cover other issues such as cultural competence, management of services to people with hearing or language difficulties, the requirement to establish written collaboration or affiliation agreements, research, interdepartmental referrals, staff travel, public relations and relationships with the media, staff development and training, and fund-raising.

Risk Management Procedures and Insurance

Health centers should have a risk management plan approved by the board that ensures that required codes are followed, property is maintained well and inspected regularly, safety activities and safety-related trainings are carried out, adequate insurances are carried, and QI information is used to help reduce organization liability.

Facilities in which health centers are located should meet all required local, state, and licensing codes, as well as Section 504 of the Rehabilitation Act of 1973 and the Americans with Disabilities Act (ADA). Certificates that codes are met and records of inspections such as those by the fire department should be kept on file. Facilities should be inspected regularly based on standards such as those used by The Joint Commission to ensure that they are clean, well maintained, and friendly and welcoming for consumers. Emergency kits and other equipment should be part of the inspections to ensure that they are fully stocked with up-to-date supplies. Also, the requirements of the Occupational Safety & Health Administration (OSHA) need to be followed regarding protecting employees from exposure to blood or other potentially infectious materials. Employees must be offered required vaccinations, and procedures must be implemented to minimize or eliminate employee exposure to blood-borne and airborne pathogens. OSHA inspectors conduct site visits of health care facilities to ensure that employers are providing safe work environments.

The risk management plan should outline the use of fire drills, mock codes, and staff training in such areas as infection control and crisis management, as well as field safety for staff who work in the community, which will be conducted at least annually. All staff need to be trained in risk management procedures, since they are the first line of defense in identifying problems that could become liabilities for the organization.

Malpractice, Negligence, and Insurance Coverage

Adequate insurance coverage is essential for any kind of health services enterprise. Three types of liability coverage must be carried: comprehensive general liability insurance for the facility and the organization; officers' and directors' liability insurance; and professional liability, or malpractice, insurance for the health care providers.

Malpractice, according to Buppert (1999), is the "failure of a professional skill that results in injury, loss, or damage," and negligence is "the prevailing legal theory of malpractice liability that includes failure to give necessary care, failure to follow up, and failure to refer when necessary." Familiarity and compliance with practice protocols and guidelines, as well as state laws, are ways of preventing lawsuits. NMHC staff should also be familiar with the state's regulations regarding the liability of the practice's collaborating physician and should know the guidelines for physicians who are required by law to collaborate with NPs regarding malpractice lawsuits based on NP negligence.

NMHCs should have collaborative practice agreements that define the joint practice roles and responsibilities of NPs and physicians working together (as cited in Brush & Capezuti, 1997). Because provider roles and responsibilities change over time, these agreements should be reviewed and updated annually to accommodate the shifting roles in the health care system. More information on such agreements can be found at www.pacode .com/secure/data/049/chapter18/subchapCtoc.html for Pennsylvania and at similar sites for other states.

Whether the NMHC is affiliated with a hospital or university will be one factor in determining the type of malpractice coverage the center should obtain for its nursing professionals. According to Buppert (1999), it is recommended that practitioners have "occurrence" insurance, which covers any incident while the health professional is insured. A "claims made" insurance policy only covers the person when the insurance policy is active, regardless of when the incident occurred. "Tail coverage" can be purchased for a period of time equivalent to the state's statute of limitations for that act of malpractice (Esposito, 2000). Other considerations are the amount of coverage and the specific acts that are covered by the insurance.

Under the Federally Supported Health Centers Assistance Act, all directly employed staff of FQHCs funded under Section 330 of the PHS Act are eligible to receive medical malpractice insurance through the Federal Tort Claim Act (FTCA) at no cost to the grantee. The intent of the FTCA was to spare funded health centers costly malpractice premiums. The center must adhere to quality assurance measures and guidelines, including a credentialing procedure for all health professionals, in order for covered professionals to be protected under this federal policy. Other health centers will need to purchase private professional liability insurance for their providers. The costs and amounts required vary from state to state. Information can be obtained at www.hpso.com.

Personnel Policies and Procedures

It is helpful to have someone on the board or available to the organization who has personnel management expertise. The board, because of their importance to an organization, must always approve personnel policies. The personnel policies should also be published in a manual that is distributed to all employees, with signatures regarding their receipt of the manual and any changes. These policies and their accompanying procedures will help the health center to manage its employees and govern its employment practices in conformity with applicable laws and regulations, including the Civil Rights Act of 1964, the Fair Labor Standards Act (as amended by the Equal Pay Act and the Age Discrimination in Employment Act), OSHA, ADA, the National Labor Relations Act, the Family and Medical Leave Act, and the Rehabilitation Act of 1973, as well as applicable state and local laws. Legal counsel should be consulted when personnel policies are developed or revised and when necessary to ensure the agency's conformity with legal requirements.

The organization should determine, through planning and budgeting, the appropriate number, qualifications, and credential requirements of the staff needed to carry out day-to-day operations and achieve the center's goals and objectives. A written position classification structure with pay ranges should be developed and used for all positions. A benefits package should also be defined, and employees should be kept informed of any changes. The organization should carry workers' compensation, payroll, and health insurance for employees in accordance with state laws and must contribute to the Federal Insurance Contributions Act (FICA) tax for all personnel. The staff eligible for medical insurance, unemployment benefits, tax-deferred accounts, and paid vacation should be determined and stated in the policy.

Job descriptions that define the experience and qualifications required for each position and that specify duties, responsibilities, and outcomes-oriented performance expectations, as well as the credentials and other requirements necessary to fulfill the job responsibilities, should be maintained for all positions. Job descriptions should clearly state how the employee's work supports the organization's mission. These are meaningful documents and should be the basis for assessing each employee's performance evaluation. Care must be taken to ensure that positions are properly classified according to federal wage and hour regulations (Free Clinic Foundation of America, 1998). Recruitment and hiring procedures should be followed to eliminate, to the degree possible, any discrimination. Established procedures and resources such as the IRS website, which provides a helpful tax guide for employers, should be used when developing hiring procedures. Legal counsel should be consulted to ensure that all requirements are met. Staffing and hiring should be reviewed regularly to ensure that the organization is adhering to the civil rights requirements of many public funders.

Procedures should be followed that ensure that all personnel receive full orientation to the organization, its policies and procedures, and the specifics of their positions. Procedures should also specify ongoing training requirements and requirements for annual employee performance reviews. It may be helpful to develop an affiliation with a health professions training institution to ensure that the latest information is available to the staff.

In order to hold personnel accountable for their responsibilities, each employee's competence to fulfill the work responsibilities described in the job description should be assessed through training evaluations and through formal performance reviews conducted at the end of the probation period and annually. Employees perform best when they are engaged in and have the tools they need to do their work and receive regular feedback from their supervisors. Employees are entitled to regular feedback from their supervisors, which should not be limited to the formal annual review, but should occur frequently and include concrete examples of each employee's success in meeting job description tasks.

FQHCs are required to conduct termination interviews with staff who leave and to use this information, and the turnover data that are tracked through the QI process, to determine if any changes need to be made to improve employee satisfaction and reduce turnover rates.

HIPAA and Information Management

Administrative policies and procedures must take into consideration the HIPAA of 1996. HIPAA was designed to protect health insurance coverage for workers and their families when they change or lose their jobs and ensure the privacy of medical information and standardized electronic data interchange. The HIPAA Standards for Privacy of Individually Identifiable Health Information, also known as the Privacy Regulations or the Privacy

Rules, are a comprehensive set of federal rules aimed at providing confidentiality protection to nearly all medical records and other individually identifiable health information. The Administrative Simplification provisions of HIPAA required that DHHS establish national standards for electronic data interchange and protection of the confidentiality and security of health data through setting and enforcing standards. More specifically, HIPAA calls for standardizing patients' electronic health, administrative, and financial data. It also requires unique health identifiers for individuals, employers, health plans, and health care providers. Finally, the act enforces security standards that protect the confidentiality and integrity of individually identifiable health information—past, present, or future.

All health care organizations, health plans, health care clearinghouses, and health care providers must be familiar with and comply with HIPAA requirements, or they face severe civil and criminal penalties ranging from fines to imprisonment. Participation in Medicare and Medicaid also requires compliance with HIPAA requirements. More information on HIPAA is available at www.hhs.gov/ocr/privacy/hipaa/understanding/index.html.

Clinical Practice Guidelines

Clinical practice guidelines are procedures that provide organized methods for analyzing and managing particular diseases or major symptoms. They ensure consistent, high-quality practice by specifying the scope of nursing practice at the health center, as well as referral mechanisms. It is recommended that a formal mechanism be put in place to update the clinical practice guidelines annually. This mechanism should be spelled out in the policies and procedures.

CONTINUOUS QUALITY/PERFORMANCE IMPROVEMENT

The health center should have a QI plan that is approved by the board and that details the philosophy, organization, scope, and methodology of the organization's QI program. This plan and its attendant procedures should specify systematic processes for monitoring and evaluating the safety, quality, and appropriateness of patient care and for identifying and resolving problems. The plan should have corresponding sections in the organization's other policies and procedures. For example, the infection control procedures should outline an effective process for monitoring their effectiveness, as should the pharmaceutical, laboratory, facility inspection, and other procedures.

The continuous QI process is enhanced by being carried out through a team structure that ensures that information gathered regarding service safety and quality is shared with, and ideas for improvement are sought from, as many staff as possible, contributing to a greater sense of ownership and responsibility.

A structure that is used in many organizations is quarterly team meetings that include all members of the staff. A representative organization-wide team that may include some board members and a management team then hold meetings where recommended actions are prioritized and approved. Other organizations impart and gather information in regular unit meetings and use a QI committee structure that involves broad representation from clinical and management staff. Minutes of all QI meetings are kept in a concise action-oriented format and are available, along with supporting materials of representative meetings, to all staff.

The QI process works with four types of information:

- Incidents, accidents, and grievances
- Peer record review and utilization review
- Stakeholder input
- Program evaluation indicators and outcomes data

This information is compiled and distributed to the teams for analysis and action. Meeting agendas consist of discussions of each type of information, QI projects, and obstacles to quality.

Incidents, Accidents, and Grievances

Analyses of incidents, accidents, and grievances provide two kinds of information and therefore are reviewed in two different ways. The study of incidents, accidents, and grievances gives the center information to use for risk management. A pattern of accidents may alert the center to a hazardous condition that should be corrected. A pattern of incidents or grievances could signal a problem that could result in lawsuits or in action by a payer. Incidents and grievances also give the center information about the quality of services being provided. A pattern of incidents may indicate to a QI team that a problem has arisen or that there is a gap in available services.

Peer Record Review and Utilization Review

Peer record reviews of current and recently closed cases can determine the extent to which health center records and the services they reflect comply with requirements and the quality of the services being provided. It also allows for an independent determination of how well services are being utilized and for monitoring resource utilization. Peer record reviews are done on statistically significant numbers of cases by staff who have not been directly involved in or directly supervised the services they are reviewing.

Stakeholder Input

Stakeholders fall into three categories: the customer/payers, such as grant-making organizations and third-party payers; the individuals and families served; and the community that the center serves, including area hospitals and specialists with which the health center works. Each team should consider how stakeholder input will be obtained, including both formal and informal ways that input and guidance may be obtained from the defined community. This input will constitute part of the needs assessment that will assist the team in reviewing the strategic plan.

Individuals can be surveyed individually or, in some instances, in groups to determine their satisfaction with the services they are receiving. Standardized survey instruments that ensure anonymity should be used where feasible.

Program Evaluation Indicators and Outcomes Data

The QI teams can use two kinds of program evaluation information. The first is the results of inspections of the services by the customer/payers, such as the state, HRSA, or The Joint Commission. One inspection is the audit carried out by the certified public accountants hired by the board each year. Problems identified in inspections should be addressed by QI projects that carry very high priority.

The second kind of program information is data gathered regarding each service in the agency. According to Kinsey and Gerrity (1997), data from health promotion, disease prevention, education, outreach, and case-finding activities should be collected, in addition to data on primary care and other services. Quantitative data are gathered, as are data selected by each QI team that can indicate the outcomes and quality of the center's services. The quantitative data indicate the numbers, demographics, and needs of the people served and the numbers and types of services provided. These data can be compared with the goals set at the beginning of each year. Teams can then determine whether numeric targets are being met or whether trends are occurring regarding the types of people receiving services. FQHCs are required to gather and review cost and productivity data; software systems are available to help with this process.

In all programs, information should be collected regarding the quality and outcomes of services. Many indicators can be found within clinical procedures, and benchmarks are set in the health care and/or strategic plan. The Bureau of Primary Health Care has also set clinical outcome measures for FQHCs that any health center can use. The benchmarks should be reviewed and revised at least annually, using the center's experience and comparing results with the experience of others who provide similar services to similar populations. Eight NMHCs in the Philadelphia area are working together on a project that is setting up a common electronic health record (EHR) and pooling outcomes data. The results of this project will begin to be available through the NNCC website in 2015.

Obstacles to Quality Service

Time can be taken at QI meetings to discuss barriers that prevent the health center from providing the highest quality services possible. These discussions might consider outside systems, such as regulators and funders, or internal processes, such as outreach, intake, assessment, and personnel or training issues.

QI Projects

Following discussion—of the QI information, what the data indicate about the services being provided, and possible explanations when the data reveal issues of concern—teams determine the QI projects to be undertaken to address the issues revealed in the data. QI projects are designed to

- Build on strengths
- Find and replicate good practices
- Eliminate or reduce identified problems
- Implement and monitor the effectiveness of the projects

INFORMATION SYSTEMS

NMHCs should have data collection systems in place so they are able to demonstrate their impact on clients served, indicate clinical outcomes, and participate in research (Barger, 1995). Data collection, particularly on patient outcomes that equate to payer cost savings, are very valuable for assisting in regulation changes in favor of independent nurse-managed practices. For example, NNCC has used cost and utilization data to make the case that NMHCs are cost-effective. These data have resulted in policy changes that have led both Medicaid and private managed care to contract with independent nursing centers.

It is important at the outset to determine what data points need to be collected and what system will be used. Additional questions to consider are what variables to enter, how much should be entered, who enters the data, who extracts the data, who will analyze the data, what data funders expect, and what system capacity and equipment are necessary. In addition to client data, the system should also track financial information related to fee collection and third-party reimbursement, as well as productivity measures for individual providers and the health center as a whole.

Elements of a practice that a health center's information systems must include are

- Billing
- Capitation management
- General ledger
- Registration/enrollment
- Scheduling
- Patient tracking
- Laboratory
- Referral tracking
- Medical records
- Pharmacy
- Word processing
- Secure messaging
- Internet access
- Spreadsheets

There are a variety of data collection systems available, the most common of which are electronic practice management (EPM) systems and EHRs. These systems are often combined in one specialized product, but may be sold separately. If an EHR/EPM solution is not an option, other electronic tracking systems may suffice, but they will lack supportive features related to networking capability and data reporting.

In addition to EPM/EHR systems, described in the following section, a business intelligence program is needed to produce custom reports and support population health management services. These programs are extremely important and helpful to NMHCs in preparing reports for providers and funders alike.

Specialized Medical Software Packages

An EPM software package consists of a number of interrelated computer programs that allow the user to schedule patient appointments, send instant messages to providers, collect and enter patients' demographic and payer information, enter clinical diagnoses and treatments performed during the visit, generate a paper or electronic bill to send to the payer, enter payments received, and track accounts receivable. Most health care providers today use an EPM because it makes office management functions much more efficient.

An EHR software package consists of a number of interrelated computer programs that enable the health care provider to collect information about patient medical history, order procedures on behalf of clients, collect outside medical information, and share medical histories with patients and outside providers. The EHR, just like the paper chart, contains information about patients' past and current medical problems and their treatments. At each visit, the provider or a member of the care team captures vital statistics such as pulse and respiration rates, blood pressure, height, weight, temperature, heart or lung sounds, results of diagnostic tests, and so on. The EHR also enables vital screening tools and allows for the collection of important personal information, such as housing and nutrition status, that affect health status. Most EHRs include clinical decision support features that remind the provider or care team member to do certain things for the patient, such as recommend that a woman have a mammogram, advise a man to have a prostate exam, or recommend that the provider administer an immunization. Once data are entered, the provider merely needs to type in the patient's name to view all of the patient's clinical information—the same kind of information that would be kept in a paper chart.

An EHR has many significant advantages:

- Information is much better organized and more readily accessible than that in a paper chart. For example, if a provider wants to see what kind of heart medication her patient has taken over the past 3 years, the EHR will display a list of both the current and past medications and their dosages.
- EHRs support care teams in the health center setting by facilitating communication between team members and allowing for standing orders. For example, an RN care manager can run a report of all the patients coming in that day who need an immunization booster. The provider can submit the order ahead of time to be filled and delivered by the medical assistant upon check-in. The provider will automatically receive a secure message from the EHR confirming that the immunization has been delivered, all before stepping into the exam room.
- Data to assess implementation of the new guidelines and patient outcomes can be extracted from the EHR database to evaluate the impact of a given change in clinical practice on patient health. For example, at the designated date or time frame, an Autochart can prompt clinicians to query a woman aged 50 or older about the date of her last mammogram, and

then provide the data entry field in which those data are entered. Similar reminder systems and decision trees for any number of clinical entities can be incorporated, as appropriate, into patient records.

- Once the EHR is implemented, it can also be used as a tool to facilitate disseminating research findings and for incorporating new practice guidelines based on those findings and agreed upon by the research infra-structure network.
- An EHR allows a health center to securely share patient data with clients, other providers (including specialists), public health registries (such as immunization directories), third-party payers, and the federal gov-ernment. In an era of increasing care coordination, these functions are necessary for participating in health networks such as accountable care organizations.
- The federal government rewards the implementation and use of EHRs through their meaningful use incentive program. Providers who serve a large number of Medicaid or Medicare clients are eligible for graduated payments if they can demonstrate the use of an EHR for data capture, data sharing, and improving clinical outcomes. These incentive pay-ments can offset a substantial portion of the cost of adopting an EHR system.

While there are many advantages of using EHR and EPM software sys-tems, there are also some disadvantages:

- These systems can be very expensive, in both initial and ongoing costs. Hardware and licenses for software must be purchased, and usually outside consultation is needed to implement new systems. Mainte-nance and purchasing of up-to-date hardware and changes in software are significant ongoing costs, as are ongoing training and training of new staff.
- Systems can become inoperable or "go down" (due to software glitches, temporary suspension of Internet service, or servers that went down). In any of these situations, clinicians and front desk staff lose their access to the application and to client data, thereby making it extremely diffi-cult to function. Some paper records may need to be maintained so that functioning can continue under these circumstances, and daily backups of the database must be performed. While server and Internet access prob-lems can be expected on occasion, software problems can be minimized by ensuring adequate staff training and selecting a vendor with an excellent reputation for customer service and support.

- Despite the promise of coordinated care across provider networks, many of the EHR systems are not interoperable, meaning they do not speak to one another without complex, expensive interface development.

To select the appropriate EHR and/or EPM systems, the health center first must decide why the product is needed. The main functions of an EPM system are front office interface (e.g., scheduling patients, scheduling providers, intraoffice communication), patient tracking, and billing software. EHRs are beneficial in that they improve documentation standardization, rapid access to specific lab results or other patient reports, and clinical decision support such as reference information regarding treatment guidelines. However, there are some barriers to EHR implementation. The health center will need a backup plan for when the system goes down and will need to convince staff members to accept the changes involved in implementation. Staff may not be computer literate and may not desire to learn these skills. In order to be considered for purchase, an EHR software product has to meet a number of criteria:

- The data entry screens must be intuitive, user-friendly, and easily navigated to encourage data entry at the point of care. They also must be structured in a manner that minimizes the possibility of data entry errors by providing drop-down lists and check boxes that eliminate or minimize the need for keystroke effort.
- Software should include already developed clinical data entry templates for the majority of common pediatric and adult examinations and clinical conditions. Behavioral health templates, while not essential, are desirable.
- The software product must be HIPAA compliant to the extent possible at the time of purchase and has to ensure HIPAA compliance because the regulations continue to be refined.
- There must be a mechanism for restricting certain client data, for example, data regarding a patient's HIV status, from view by unauthorized staff.
- The EHR vendor must be fiscally sound, with continual growth in profits and a substantial ongoing investment in product research and development, thereby increasing the likelihood that it will remain in business and be able to support the software system.
- Data entered in the EHR software must be capable of being exported in a file format that can be read by statistical software such as the Statistical Package for the Social Sciences (SPSS) or the Statistical Analysis System (SAS).

- Data entry templates and data fields in the EHR must be modifiable to be consistent with the variable definitions and levels specified by clinical research and reporting protocols.
- The system must allow for sharing patient data through a variety of means, including electronic patient portals, between provider organizations, and with public health registry programs.
- The cost of buying into the system and the annual maintenance and support costs needs to be affordable for low-budget, nonprofit nursing centers.
- The software company must have a reputation for excellent customer support and utilize a deployment system that requires minimal maintenance.

The health center will need to establish guidelines to detail medical record maintenance, access to records, consent requirements for release of information, and exceptions to those consent requirements, as well as procedures to ensure the confidentiality of patients' medical records that comply with HIPAA provisions. Procedures should also indicate security measures, backup procedures, and requirements that backups be stored off-site, as well as a disaster plan in case the facility is destroyed or there is system failure.

Fortunately for health centers, there is a plethora of support materials to help them evaluate the costs and benefits associated with EHR adoption. The federal government's Office of the National Coordinator for Health Information Technology (ONCHIT) maintains a list of certified EHR products that meet rigorous requirements related to data security, clinical features, and reporting capability. The full list of ONCHIT-certified products can be found at http://oncchpl.force.com/ehrcert/CHPLHome. Additionally, ONCHIT maintains a library of documents to help health centers evaluate potential EHR vendor companies, develop an EHR implementation plan, and optimize the use of an EHR to support quality care. ONCHIT's toolkit is accessible at www.healthit.gov/providers-professionals/implementation-resources.

REFERENCES

Adams, C. M. (2002, January 8). Building credibility with grantmakers. *Charity Channel LLC, 1*(15).

Barger, S. E. (1995). Establishing a nursing center: Learning from the literature and the experiences of others. *Journal of Professional Nursing, 11*(4), 203–212. doi: 10.1016/S8755-7223(95)80021-2

Brush, B. L., & Capezuti, E. A. (1997). Professional autonomy: Essential for nurse practitioner survival in the 21st century. *Journal of the American Academy of Nurse Practitioners, 9*(6), 265–270. doi: 10.1111/j.1745-7599.1997.tb00718.x

Buppert, C. (1999). *Nurse practitioner's business practice and legal guide*. Gaithersburg, MD: Aspen Publication.

Clemen-Stone, S., McGuire, S. L., & Eigsti, D. G. (2002). *Comprehensive community health nursing: Family, aggregate, & community practice* (6th ed.). Philadelphia, PA: Mosby.

Dunphy, L. M. H. (Ed.). (1999). *Management guidelines for adult nurse practitioners*. Philadelphia, PA: F. A. Davis.

Elsberry, N., & Nelson, F. (1993). How to plan financial support for nursing centers. *Nursing & Health Care, 14*(8), 408–413.

Esposito, C. L. (2000). What's the point of malpractice insurance? *Nursing Spectrum, 12*(13), 6–7.

Fazzano, M. L. (2002). *Getting on the radar: How to approach family foundations*. Retrieved from http://www.changingourworld.com/index.html

Free Clinic Foundation of America, Inc. (1998). *A free clinic: Starting out*. Roanoke, VA: Author.

Glick, D. F., Hale, P. J., Kulbok, P. A., & Shettig, J. (1996). Community development theory: Planning a community nursing center. *Journal of Nursing Administration, 26*(7), 44–50. doi: 10.1097/00005110-199607000-00010

Hansen-Turton, T., Greiner, P., Miller, M. E., & Deinhardt, A. (Eds.). (2009). *Nurse-managed wellness centers: Developing and maintaining your center*. New York, NY: Springer Publishing.

Kinsey, K. K., & Gerrity, P. (1997). Planning, implementing, and managing a community-based nursing center: Current challenges and future opportunities. In M. Harris (Ed.), *Handbook of home health care administration* (2nd ed.). New York, NY: Aspen Publishers.

Lundeen, S. P. (1999). An alternative paradigm for promoting health in communities: The Lundeen community nursing center model. *Family & Community Health, 21*(4), 15–28. doi: 10.1097/00003727-199901000-00004

CHAPTER 4

Nurse-Managed Health Centers and Sustainability

Bonita Ann Pilon and Tine Hansen-Turton

STRATEGIES FOR SUSTAINING NURSE-MANAGED CLINICS: A BALANCING ACT

The most recent Health Resources and Services Administration (HRSA) National Sample Survey of Nurse Practitioners (2014, p. 3) reported that there are more than 132,000 nurse practitioners (NPs) in the U.S. workforce working in positions that require an NP credential. Over 127,000 provide direct patient care, and nearly half of those (60,407) are working in primary care. The settings for practice vary widely from private physician offices to hospitals. Of particular interest are those NPs who report practicing in private NP office practices and in nurse-managed clinics ($N = 5,649$). This chapter focuses on methods and strategies for financial sustainability in NP practices and nurse-managed health clinics (NMHCs).

At the end of this chapter, the reader will be able to

- Describe common approaches to financial stability for NMHCs and private practices
- Determine the key variables to consider when evaluating a capitation contract

- Analyze the results of operations to determine where adjustments can be made to increase the sustainability of the practice or clinic
- Describe two non-fee-for-service (non-FFS) sources of funding for NMHCs and private practices

The Most Common Approaches to Financial Stability

There are three prevalent models for creating revenue to sustain a nurse-managed, community-based practice: fee for service, contract, and grant. Each model is discussed in the following text.

The FFS Model

Health care providers have traditionally been paid through an FFS model. This approach, while still prevalent, is likely to shift—perhaps dramatically—over the next 5 years. The key elements of the FFS model include a fee schedule set by the provider and linked to Current Procedural Terminology (CPT) and International Classification of Diseases (ICD)-9/10 codes; contracts between the provider and the various health insurance plans that stipulate the discounted payment rates for services rendered to their enrollees; a billing system that can receive claims submitted electronically; a contract with an electronic claims clearinghouse; and a discounted fee schedule for patients who pay for their own care (uninsured).

This model has been the foundation for payment for all clinical encounters in community private practice since physicians made horse-and-buggy rounds and were paid with chickens, eggs, fruits, and vegetables raised by the farmer who received care. As medical care became more sophisticated and as the population shifted from farms to cities, cash became the mode of transaction. In the late 1930s and throughout the 1940s, the notion of health insurance became more dominant, and when Medicare and Medicaid were enacted in 1966, provider payments moved almost exclusively into the claims system rather than direct payment from the patient.

In order to effectively (and exclusively) use an FFS model to sustain a private NP practice or NMHC, the payer mix must be understood and analyzed. Payer mix refers to the volume of patients from each health plan (including Medicare and Medicaid) that are projected to be treated by the NP provider during any given period. Most practices project their mixes for 12 months when creating a budget for the coming year; however, the mix must be evaluated each month during the year to determine if the patient volume is matching the prediction (see Table 4.1).

Note that in this NP practice, the projected number of Blue Cross Blue Shield (BCBS) and commercial patient encounters decreased by 700 visits,

Table 4.1 Nurse-Led Clinic Payer Mix Analysis: Patient Visits

Payer	Budgeted Volume	Actual Volume	Variance
BCBS	2,500	2,100	(400)
Commercial	1,500	1,200	(300)
Medicare	1,000	1,150	150
Medicaid	2,800	2,798	(2)
Self-pay	1,500	1,600	100

BCBS, Blue Cross Blue Shield.

while Medicare and self-pay volume increased by a total of 250 visits. This shift likely had a negative impact on the bottom line, as the next two tables illustrate. In Table 4.2, the actual revenue per visit is compared with the budgeted amount. This clinic projected, through the use of available data that included the contract signed with each payer and historical data at this setting, that BCBS patients would on average bring in $75 per visit; the actual collections were higher, $76 per visit. For commercial patients, the practice also did better on their collections, and they collected more per patient from Medicare. However, self-pay patients' per-visit collections decreased by $9 per visit. Medicaid actually increased, but not enough to offset the self-pay losses. These per-visit differences may not make a substantial difference in the bottom line for this practice—it depends on *how many of each type* of patient were actually seen. See Table 4.3 to discover the impact on revenue when the *patient volume* and *patient revenue per visit* per payer type change.

In Table 4.3, the variance between what the practice expected to collect and what it actually collected is negative (down $25,130). During this period, even though the collections per patient visit were higher for BCBS,

Table 4.2 Nurse-Led Clinic Revenue per Visit Analysis

Payer	Budgeted Revenue per Visit	Actual	Variance
BCBS	$75.00	$76.00	$1.00
Commercial	$83.00	$85.00	$2.00
Medicare	$54.00	$65.00	$11.00
Medicaid	$35.00	$40.00	$5.00
Self-pay	$50.00	$41.00	($9.00)

BCBS, Blue Cross Blue Shield.

Table 4.3 Nurse-Led Clinic Payer Mix Analysis: Revenue

Payer	Budgeted Collections	Actual Collections	Variance
BCBS	$187,500.00	$159,600.00	($27,900.00)
Commercial	$124,500.00	$102,000.00	($22,500.00)
Medicare	$54,000.00	$74,750.00	$20,750.00
Medicaid	$98,000.00	$111,920.00	$13,920.00
Self-pay	$75,000.00	$65,600.00	($9,400.00)
Total	**$539,000.00**	**$513,870.00**	**$25,130.00**

BCBS, Blue Cross Blue Shield.

commercial insurance, Medicare, and Medicaid, the volumes of BCBS and commercial patients were lower than expected, and the resulting collections were down by a combined $50,400. This shortfall heavily influenced the variance from budget. (The increased collections for Medicare and Medicaid were not enough to offset the losses from the two other payers.) A budget is a plan, and for this particular plan, the money collected did not match expectations. When that happens, there are only two possible solutions for keeping the practice open: Reduce expenses to match the shortfall (the expense budget is discussed later in the chapter), or find other funding to cover the collections shortfall. The source of additional funds could be cash that was already in the bank or it could be a loan. These are immediate solutions to cash short-falls, but there are other possible solutions that will take longer to develop: Renegotiate the payer contract to increase the pay rate (this can be difficult, but it should not be overlooked); seek other NP businesses that are not paid on an FFS, volume basis; or consider becoming an "owned practice" by a larger system that needs NP services within its network and believes that this practice would add value to its mission and bottom line. For this latter strategy, the NP would become an employee of the larger system, and the practice's revenue would flow directly to the new entity.

This case example illustrates the challenges in a pure FFS model. Across the country among physician primary care practices, an increasing number are facing shortfalls just like this one, and many are opting to become employed. In 2013, Becker Hospital Review reported that the number of employed primary care physicians had risen to 40%, double the previous number, and was projected to continue to rise, particularly among younger physicians. According to 2010 data from the Medical Group Management Association, 65% of physicians already in practice who changed jobs and

49% of those who had just completed their residencies took positions in hospital-based practices in 2009 (Elliot, 2011). This shift of physicians from independent private practice to employed status reflects the cost-versus-revenue challenges they face. NP private practices and NMHCs face the same revenue challenges, and the costs of practice are similar, with the exception of NP salary and malpractice costs. Running an office practice costs the same regardless of the provider; salaries and malpractice costs vary, but not, for example, the costs of the building, support staff, and utilities. Given the trend in physician private practice, will NP private practice follow? Or will fewer NPs choose to establish private, nurse-managed clinic models? Trends over the next 5 years will be interesting to watch.

One possible alternative to leaving private practice is allowing NP providers to contract with payers to accept capitation payments for covered lives. Capitation contracts can be in addition to standard FFS contracts, as is illustrated here. Capitation is attractive in that there is a steady flow of dollars to the practice each month, regardless of whether any patients are actually seen. However, capitation rates and responsibilities must be carefully examined to determine if this type of FFS will produce a positive cash flow for the practice.

Capitation rates are the dollars per patient (member) per month (PMPM) that the payer is willing to pay the provider for a set of services that enrollees who are assigned to the provider for their medical home will receive. More assigned patients increase the amount of money that the provider receives each month. Usually, the primary care provider (PCP) is responsible for all preventative care and chronic illness management and may be financially responsible for care coordination with specialists as well. The devil is in the details: Providers should negotiate lab and other diagnostic tests as a "carve-out" so that they are not responsible for paying those costs from their capitation payments. Capitation can be a windfall for providers, but it can also be a financial risk depending on the terms offered. In the example depicted in Table 4.4, the capitation rates do not include any practice expenses for diagnostic testing; those expenses were carved out of the capitation contracts signed by the provider, and the budget must be adjusted whenever the provider's financial risk changes. Hopefully, if the NP provider is expected to provide additional services, the capitation rate will be higher than that depicted here. All of the examples for this practice are for illustrative purposes only: Each NP practice must consider all of the variables, including contract rates, actual cost of practice, services to be rendered, and changing market conditions, in order to accurately predict both expenses and revenue.

Table 4.4 Capitation Revenue Projections

Payer	Number Assigned Lives	PMPM	Budgeted Revenue
Medicaid MCO	500	$12.00	$72,000.00
Alliance MCO	500	$15.00	$90,000.00
HealthOne MCO	500	$18.00	$108,000.00
Medicare Advantage	500	$28.00	$168,000.00
		Total	$438,000.00

MCO, Managed care organization; PMPM, Per patient (member) per month.

The table shows the number of assigned lives per managed care organization (MCO) in this NP practice. The PMPM payment varies among the payers, and this is generally true in all markets, with Medicaid MCOs having the lowest PMPM. Note that this NP contracted to take 500 lives from each of the payers, for a total of 2,000 assigned lives. For each capitation contract, this NP assumed responsibility for these patients' primary care. The patients were able to schedule visits at any time during the budget year, and the NP had to meet contract performance requirements with regard to timely appointments and medical management according to national guidelines. Medical home accountability is built into each contract, so the NP and staff must plan for all of the care coordination and wraparound services required to keep these patients functioning at their optimal levels of wellness, as spelled out in the capitation contract. Each contract will differ by the payer's expectations for levels of responsibility and accountability.

Revenue from these contracts will bring in an additional $438,000 per budget period to this practice. Previously, the NP clinic had more than $25,000 in losses from the traditional FFS revenue (Table 4.3). With the addition of $438,000 in revenue, this clinic now shows a positive collections variance of $412,870. In this case, the capitation contracts seem to have helped stabilize and sustain the practice and created a large surplus. However, the expense budget must also be examined to be certain (see Table 4.5).

The expense budget was built based on the expected patient volume. Table 4.5 displays the annual budget. Earlier data (Tables 4.1 and 4.3) show that this practice experienced 8,848 FFS and self-pay patient visits. Table 4.4 shows a total of 2,000 patients assigned through capitation arrangements. In order to determine the practice's staffing budget—the most expensive component of practice—certain assumptions must be made. For the budget in Table 4.5, these assumptions were made:

Table 4.5 NP Practice Expense Budget

	Expense	
Salaries	(2.5 NPs, 3 MAs, 3 registration clerks, 1 LPN, 1 RN)	$496,000.00
Benefits	@26%	$128,960.00
Rent	(3,000 sq. ft.)	$54,000.00
Utilities		$4,800.00
Insurance	(medical malpractice, general liability)	$6,500.00
Supplies		$126,432.00
Equipment		$5,000.00
EMR		$12,600.00
Billing	10% of collections	$95,187.00
Total Expenses		**$929,479.00**

EMR, electronic medical record; LPN, licensed practice nurse; MA, medical assistant; NP, nurse practitioner.

- The practice is open 50 weeks per year.
- Currently, there are 8,848 FFS visits, divided by 50, which equals an average of 177 patients per week or 35 per day.
- Two thousand capitation patients will visit the clinic at an average of 2.6 visits per patient per year (national estimates range from 1.8 to 3.32).
- Capitation patient visit volume equals 2,000 × 2.6, or 5,200 additional visits per year.
- Ideal PCP panel size ranges from 1,387 to 1,947 (Altschuler, Margolius, Bodenheimer, & Grumbach, 2012); in this practice, panel size is 800 per provider because there are over 8,000 other visits per year from noncapitation patients whom the advanced practice registered nurses (APRNs) must also manage.
- The total estimated patient visits per year equal 8,848 + 5,200, or 14,048.
- Total patient visits per week equals 281.
- Total patient visits per day (5-day work week) equals 56.
- Supplies are assumed to be $9 per patient encounter (14,048 × $9).

Given the high volume of patients per day/week/year, the practice budgets for 2.5 NP PCPs, three medical assistants, three registration clerks, one licensed practice nurse (LPN), and one registered nurse (RN). The ratio of NP provider to support staff is 1:3.2. Billing personnel are not included in these calculations because it is assumed that the clinic will contract with an outside billing company to handle all billing and collection activities. The practice budget estimates that billing services will cost 10% of each dollar collected, and that expense is included in Table 4.5. In this example, the ratio of provider to support staff is an average based on national standards. The U.S. Department of Veterans Affairs reported that three support staff to one PCP was required for a successful medical home model (2012). NMHCs have traditionally been less well staffed than their physician counterparts, many times because of their propensity to serve vulnerable populations, for which the revenue potential is less robust. In this case example, the NP practice is serving all payers from self-pay to Medicaid, private insurance plans, and Medicare.

With traditional FFS revenue of $513,870 and capitation collections of $438,000, does this NP practice make enough money to cover its expenses, as depicted in Table 4.5? Total revenue/collections are $951,870 versus total expenses of $929,479, so this practice currently has a profit of $22,391. Adding the capitation contracts not only enabled this practice to overcome its previous shortfall, but also created a positive cash flow. Note that the practice had to employ a number of support personnel in order to meet the capitation contract demands. Medical home services require active care coordination by the provider in order to fulfill the terms of most capitation contracts. The RN is likely to spend the majority of her or his time assisting patients to navigate primary and specialist care. Follow-up phone calls, responding to electronic health record (EHR) patient portal interactivity, and proactive outreach for prevention are hallmarks of a well-executed capitation agreement. In a busy practice like this one, additional staff are required for both clinical and financial success.

Table 4.6 shows the estimated revenue per visit for capitated patients. This is only an estimate; at the end of the budget period, the NP practice must compare the actual number of visits by capitated patients to determine how much revenue was actually realized. If these projections are accurate, it is apparent that revenue from capitation patients is higher per visit than

Table 4.6 Capitation Revenue per Encounter

Payer	Lives	Visits per Patient	PMPM	Revenue per Visit
Medicaid MCO	500	2.6	$12.00	$55.38
Alliance MCO	500	2.6	$15.00	$69.23
HealthOne MCO	500	2.6	$18.00	$83.08
Medicare Advantage	500	2.6	$28.00	$129.23

MCO, managed care organization; PMPM, per patient (member) per month.

revenue from many of the FFS patients. In a capitation arrangement, the provider holds financial risk: If there are more patient visits than projected, the provider spends more of the capitation money to provide services; if there are fewer visits than projected, the provider keeps more of the capitation money as profit. The contract terms guard against any failure to provide needed clinical services by specifying the clinical and efficiency performance metrics that must be met.

If capitation contracts were not available or were not sufficient to close the gap between expenses and collections, what other strategies might be useful in closing this gap? Renegotiating the payment rates with payers is one strategy, but for Medicare and Medicaid plans, these rates are regional or national and will be very unlikely to change. Private insurers have more leeway to increase prices, but the trend has been going the other way: PCPs have seen rate reductions in the past several years, and provider incomes have been falling, so this strategy does not seem like the easiest or fastest solution to the problem. As demonstrated in the discussion here, a microanalysis of the payer mix is likely to lead to better decision making for the NP practice.

If the practice had elected to not participate in any capitation contracts—or none were available—both the expense budget and the revenue would be reduced. Would these changes be enough to create a positive bottom line? See the new expense budget in Table 4.7, now that the capitation contracts are no longer included. Eliminating these contracts results in an expense budget

Table 4.7 NP Practice Expense Budget Without Cap Contracts

Expense		
Salaries/Benefits	(1.5 NPs, 2 MAs, 1 registration clerk, 1 LPN)	$321,300.00
Rent	(2,000 sq. ft.)	$36,000.00
Utilities		$3,000.00
Insurance	(medical malpractice, general liability)	$4,500.00
Supplies		$79,632.00
Equipment		$3,000.00
EMR		$10,600.00
Billing	10% of collections	$51,387.00
Total Expenses		**$509,419.00**

EMR, electronic medical record; LPN, licensed practice nurse; MA, medical assistant; NP, nurse practitioner.

that is $4,451 *less* than the actual collections—these dollars are profit for the NMHC. The staffing model was adjusted to 1.5 full-time equivalent (FTE) NPs and 1.0 clerk to reflect the reduced number of visits to the practice (5,200 fewer visits when there are no capitation patients in the payer mix), and the supply budget was also adjusted for fewer patient encounters. The practice is projected to see 35 patients per day rather than the 56 in the earlier scenario.

Every market is different, and the NP practice must periodically reassess the local market and adjust both the revenue and expense budgets to reflect changing conditions. *Proactive planning and analysis are absolutely critical to remaining fiscally viable.*

The Contract Model

A second model for ensuring the financial stability of NP private practices and NMHCs involves contracting to provide certain clinical services, ranging from urgent or episodic care to full primary care, for a defined patient population. The most prevalent populations served in these models are university students (student health services) and employer health sites. There can be myriad other contractual arrangements depending on the local market and on the entrepreneurial skills of the NP provider. These contracts are not third-party payer contracts; they are private contracts between the NP practice entity and the agency that desires the services for its population.

A number of student health services, at both small colleges and major universities, are managed by the nursing school faculty practice programs under contracts or internal memoranda of agreement between the university and the school. Such contracts generally do not have a profit motive, meaning that the school does not mark up its cost to provide these services in order to gain profits itself. There is often, however, an indirect cost applied to the agreement that allows the nursing school to realize a small amount of the recouped costs that are incurred for overseeing these clinical services. The direct costs for all of the providers, support personnel, supplies, equipment, EHRs, insurance, and so on are paid by the university. The clinic may or may not bill the student's third-party payer—this is a school's decision, and some universities do not attempt to bill because they consider student health services to be part of their student services and paid for by student fees. Other universities may charge a small cash fee for students to be seen. Each situation is unique.

There are several benefits to the school and to the faculty and staff who provide these primary and episodic care services. Faculty have an established practice venue where they can remain clinically active and maintain their national board certification requirements. These clinics also provide possible student primary care placement sites for advanced practice nursing students. There may be an opportunity to offer behavioral health services that engage additional advanced practice faculty members in practice. Funding for these practice sites is essentially guaranteed from year to year, and if a university changes its plan for staffing the student health center, there should be ample time for the school of nursing to plan an exit strategy.

Employer on-site and near-site episodic and primary care clinics are a growing phenomenon. The most recent Mercer survey in 2012 reported that 32% to 37% of companies with 5,000 or more employees had an on-site clinic, and an additional 15% of companies in this category were considering opening one. For smaller employers (500–4,999 employees), 15% had an on-site clinic, and another 11% were planning to open one in the next 12 to 15 months (Mercer, 2012 as cited in Anderson, 2013). These companies comprise nearly one third of the employers (30%) that now offer on-site clinics to their workers. Twenty-six percent of clinics in companies with over 500 employees focused on occupational health; however, the interest in clinics is expanding to include primary care. Often companies are not sure what scopes of service best fit their needs. NPs can be quite valuable in working with employers to help them define the services that meet their goals in opening an on-site clinic. The most prevalent reasons reported by Mercer were to reduce lost employee productivity (82%), decrease the employer's overall health care spending (75%), and provide a benefit that retains employees (47%; Anderson, 2013). From a long-term perspective, employer clinics can improve overall employee health and thus decrease the employer's costs.

Serving as a near-site clinic may be useful to an NP private practice or NMHC. For example, the NP practice could work with an employer to locate an office practice very near the worksite, and this clinic could function as a regular practice site that serves all types of patients who want to establish a medical home. In addition, the clinic could contract to receive and treat any employee and/or dependent during regular clinic hours, and the clinic would be paid a set price per contract for these services. In this scenario, the NP clinic will likely have a time frame within which staff must comply to see patients and return them to work. For example, the contract may stipulate that company patients be seen within 10 minutes of arrival, limiting any wait time. The NP will need to plan workflow to accommodate the possible influx of these patients throughout the day. The employer will likely want all Department of Transportation (DOT) physicals to be performed by the NP, and therefore the providers will need to take the mandatory DOT training, pass the exam, and be listed on the National Registry in order to perform this contracted service. Occupational health services may be included in the contract as well. Annual flu immunizations for workers and perhaps their dependents may be included. There are myriad possible episodic, preventive, occupational, and primary care services that could be included in a contract. Both the employer and the NP clinic must take time to discern what set of services best fits the employer's needs as well as the clinic's capacity to deliver those services.

These contracts generally have generous profit margins built in, but again, the devil is in the details. The NP practice must adequately plan its expenses based on the services to be offered and the projected patient volume. There should be a provision in the contract for amending services or for increasing payments under specified conditions such as increased volume; if the volume of care increases beyond a certain level, the NP practice will have increased costs, and those costs need to be passed back to the employer. Particularly in the first 2 years of a new employer arrangement, the utilization patterns will be difficult to project, and to protect both the NP practice and the employer, the ability to amend the contract terms is imperative.

There are many other contract opportunities for NP practices to both supplement their incomes and provide community benefit. Seasonal flu immunization campaigns are generally an easy way to work with local non-profit agencies and provide high visibility within the community. These agencies hire the nurse-managed clinic to provide the flu vaccine to a specific population, and the vaccine and medication administration costs are paid for by the agency. Small contracts like these often lead to other requests for services as the relationship grows. In addition, the positive publicity from such events raises the public's awareness of the NP practice, creating goodwill and expanding the markets for potential clinic patients.

The Grant Model

The third approach to funding NMHCs and NP practices is grants. Grants are monies awarded, usually after a competitive review process, to organizations for a specific purpose. For example, the HRSA Division of Nursing regularly issues requests for proposals (RFPs) for nurse-centric clinical work, and a number of those RFPs over the past 30 years have been targeted toward nurse-managed clinics and NP practices. These grants have supported the development and expansion of many NMHCs across the country, and many of these have been developed and managed by schools of nursing. Another very important federal source of grant funding is the HRSA Bureau of Primary Care, from which the federally qualified health center (FQHC) program is administered. Periodically, this bureau issues RFPs for New Starts—new applications for FQHCs. All federal grant programs are highly competitive with limited funding.

Private foundation grants are another potential source of funding for nurse-managed care. National foundations such as the United Health Foundation and Aetna Foundation usually have set agendas during each year for which they seek applicants to fulfill their objectives. These RFPs are competitive, and applicants submit nationally. The scope of services requested may be focused locally or may encompass regional, state, or national goals. The NP practice must carefully read the RFP to determine whether the stated objectives of the foundation match well with the clinic's capacity to meet the objectives.

Local or regional foundations can be quite valuable to a nurse-managed clinic. These foundations are engaged in their local communities and have a much greater awareness of the work of the NMHCs in their areas than do national foundations or federal agencies. Reputation for community service is a valuable commodity when a grant proposal is reviewed. These local foundations almost always restrict their funding to smaller grants that target a specific need within the community. For example, a local foundation may respond positively to a proposal for supplemental funding to do outreach to the city's homeless population. The clinic might request $50,000 per year for 3 years in order to send a part-time NP to the local homeless shelter several times per week to provide primary care. The proposal might include outcome measures to determine the impact on the population who received the care. Simple measures could include the following: number of unique patients, number of patient visits, major diagnoses (ICD-9/10), pre- and posttest self-efficacy scores, specialist referrals needed, specialist referrals obtained, prescription drugs needed, prescriptions actually filled, and so on. These latter statistics build the foundation for a second grant request for funding to provide the patients with specialist care and medications.

Grants are an invaluable source of funding for NP practices and clinics. However, they are time limited, and they almost never provide complete funding for any project. And grant writing takes time and research. To be effective in leveraging grant funding for NP practices, keep these "rules" in mind when reviewing an RFP:

- Be sure that the NP practice's capacity matches the grant requirements. Stretching capacity by using the funding is okay, but be sure that the clinic will be able to continue to perform all other work without additional burdens that are not funded by the grant.

- Pay attention to budget detail when preparing the proposal. Do not underestimate the cost to perform the services required by the grant terms.
- Write proposals for work that fits very well into the practice's overall mission and vision. For example, if the clinic is a primary care site now, is there capacity to add midwifery or behavioral health? If not, should the clinic submit a proposal for a grant that requires these additional services?
- Grants are time limited. How will this grant-supported service be sustained once external funding ends? What will happen to patients who are acquired as part of the grant?
- Do not underestimate the time burden for grant reporting. Periodic reports will be required including budget analysis and results, clinical data analysis, and a narrative to describe progress toward objectives.

All NP practices and nurse-managed clinics should routinely scan the environment for federal, state, and local grant opportunities. These can provide the catalyst for expanding services that the practice hoped to accomplish at some future date. Using external dollars to jump-start the vision is strategic when vision, capacity, and funding opportunity are well aligned.

Sources for grants include www.grants.gov (federal) and www.foundationcenter.org (private foundations). The former is a public database website; the latter requires a subscription fee for full access to its extensive database.

Alternate and Novel Funding Sources

A new approach to solving society's problems through capital infusion is developing in the United States. According to Social Finance US, this new approach is called impact investing, and it uses social impact bonds (SIBs). These were first introduced in the United Kingdom in 2010 and have just begun to spread within the United States. SIBs are designed to raise capital to expand successful social programs, and health is included in the definition of social programming (Social Finance US, 2014). All parties benefit from SIB funding: Cash-strapped governments gain the flexibility to launch and sustain prevention programs; social and health service providers receive long-term sustained funding to help them implement and document programs that produce a positive return on investment; investors receive a positive gain while improving society; and service providers receive the highest quality support to achieve evidence-based outcomes (Social Finance US, 2014).

One health care example is underway in Fresno, California: In April 2013, Social Finance US and Collective Health launched an asthma management demonstration project. This 2-year project is designed to prove the effectiveness of up-front investment in asthma management by focusing on solid evidence and performance measurement. Fresno has a high rate of pediatric asthma; 20% of children have been diagnosed with the disease, which has a high impact on poor communities. Two service providers, the Central California Asthma Collaborative and Clínica Sierra Vista, work with the families of 200 low-income children with asthma to provide home care, education, and support in reducing environmental triggers ranging from cigarette smoke to dust mites. Social Finance expects that the program will produce meaningful cost savings and quality-of-life improvement for the children. There are rigorous data collection and analysis procedures embedded in the project. This is the first health-focused SIB for this funder (Social Finance US, 2014).

In describing what social issues are best suited for this financial approach, Social Finance (www.socialfinanceus.org/faqs) stated the following:

> While initial interest in SIBs focused on prison recidivism and homelessness as two promising areas, it is evident that SIBs may be deployed in a variety of additional issue areas. Some promising areas include health care (aging in place, management of chronic illnesses); early childhood education; adult education and workforce skills for hard-to-employ individuals; and nurse home-visiting programs.

NPs may benefit from the evolution of this new financial focus on positive social impact, particularly since many NMHCs and NP practices focus their work on vulnerable populations. NPs have well-established expertise in chronic illness management, aging in place, and nurse home visit programs that should position them well to become service providers for health-related programs funded using SIBs.

CONCLUSION

Financial sustainability for any clinical practice is challenging. NPs and NMHCs face many of the same market issues as physicians, and they also face additional challenges related to payer enrollment (e.g., payer bias against APRN providers) and state overregulation of practice (supervision rules). These latter two challenges can additionally impact the financial viability of nurse-managed care by altering the available payer mix (fewer commercially insured patients; more Medicaid and self-pay patients) and by adding cost to the practice (payment to physicians for required oversight). It is critically important that NPs actively explore additional and nontraditional funding streams. This chapter described several successful contract approaches as well as the advantages of public and private grants to support APRN practices and clinics. Also discussed was an emerging funding stream, very new in the United States, that may create opportunities for advanced practice nurses, particularly those whose practices are focused on vulnerable and disenfranchised populations.

REFERENCES

Altschuler, J., Margolius, D., Bodenheimer, T., & Grumbach, K. (2012). Estimating a reasonable patient panel size for primary care physicians with team-based delegation. *Annals of Family Medicine, 10*(5), 396–400. doi:10.1370/afm.1400

Anderson, C. (2013, March 13). *More large employers adding onsite health clinics.* Retrieved from http://www.healthcarefinancenews.com/news/more-large-employers-adding-site-health-clinics

Elliot, V. S. (2011, June 27). Small practices: Adapting to survive. *American Medical News.* Retrieved from http://www.amednews.com/article/20110627/business/306279969/4/

Health Resources and Services Administration National Center for Health Workforce Analysis. (2014). *Highlights from the 2012 national sample survey of nurse practitioners.* Rockville, MD. Retrieved from http://bhpr.hrsa.gov/healthworkforce/supplydemand/nursing/nursepractitionersurvey/npsurveyhighlights.pdf

Social Finance US. (2014). *Asthma management demonstration project in Fresno, CA paves way for social impact bond.* Boston, MA. Retrieved from http://socialfinanceus.org/sites/socialfinanceus.org/files/Fresno%20Asthma%20Demonstration%20Project%20Press%20Release.pdf

U.S. Department of Veterans Affairs, Veterans Health Administration. (2012). *Federal patient-centered medical home (PCMH) collaborative: Catalogue of federal PCMH activities as of October 2012.* Retrieved from http://pcmh.ahrq.gov/sites/default/files/attachments/VA_PCMH_Activities_Public_Final(1).pdf

CHAPTER 5

The Role of the Collaborative Team in Nurse-Managed Health Centers

Nancy L. Rothman and Donald B. Parks

CRNPs: LEADING INTERDISICIPLINARY/INTERPROFESSIONAL COLLABORATIVE TEAMS

Nurse-managed health centers (NMHCs) function as interdisciplinary/ interprofessional collaborative teams, with certified registered nurse practitioners (CRNPs) leading the team. Currently, state regulations vary and determine whether a CRNP can function autonomously or is required to have a supervisory or collaborative physician. It should be noted that the Institute of Medicine promotes nurses as full partners with physicians in redesigning health care in the United States (2010). Collaborative teams are consistent with patient-centered and primary care medical homes. The literature supports improved patient outcomes with interdisciplinary collaboration.

NMHC interdisciplinary/interprofessional collaborative teams may include nurse practitioners (NPs); supervisory or collaborating physicians in family medicine, pediatrics, internal medicine, and psychiatry; specialty physicians (e.g., cardiologists, podiatrists); RNs; medical assistants; medical receptionists; behavioral health counselors; psychologists; social workers; and referral managers. In addition, there are administrative positions that oversee fiscal management, operations, and quality.

Models for Collaborative Practice

Merriam-Webster defines *collaboration* as working together, especially in a joint intellectual effort. The Interprofessional Education Collaborative Expert Panel in 2011 identified core competencies in four specific areas that health care providers should employ to ensure effective interprofessional collaborative practice:

- Values/Ethics for Interprofessional Practice
  - *Work with individuals from other professions to maintain a climate of mutual respect and shared values.*
- Roles/Responsibilities
  - *Use the knowledge of one's own role and those of other professions to appropriately assess and address the health care needs of the patients and populations served.*
- Interprofessional Communication
  - *Communicate with patients, families, communities, and other health professionals in a responsive and responsible manner that supports a team approach to maintaining health and treating disease.*
- Teams and Teamwork
  - *Apply relationship-building values and the principles of team dynamics to perform effectively in different team roles to plan and deliver patient- and population-centered care that is safe, timely, efficient, effective, and equitable.*

Collaborative teams need to understand the roles of all team members and value each one's expertise. Recognition that collaborative patient care is a shared responsibility promotes interdisciplinary communication and teamwork toward enhanced patient outcomes while reducing health care costs (Somers, Marton, Barbaccia, & Randolph, 2000; Taliani, Bricker, Adelman, Cronholm, & Gabbay, 2013; Taylor, Oberle, Crutcher, & Norton, 2005).

Drummond, Abbot, Williamson, and Somji (2012) reported on successfully using the D'Amour and Oandasan (2004) model, commissioned by Health Canada, to evaluate interprofessional collaboration. This model comprises four factors: (a) shared goals and vision, including communication and shared decision making; (b) a sense of belonging, requiring trust in the expertise of others on the team and a willingness to collaborate; (c) governance, indicating the need for leadership support for interprofessional collaboration and leadership on site with the use of both formal and informal team meetings (e.g., huddles); and (d) structuring clinical care to include collegial development of protocols, practice manuals, and procedures.

Highly successful interdisciplinary/interprofessional NMHC teams incorporate the core competencies and factors introduced in the preceding text. The organizations have mission statements that all staff understand and support. The mission statement is addressed in the performance evaluations of staff in all organizational roles. All staff roles have job descriptions available so others can both understand and appreciate the expertise as well as the boundaries of the roles. Both formal and informal communication are encouraged to ensure shared decision making among staff with a broad range of expertise. There is interdisciplinary/interprofessional team involvement in all clinical, fiscal, operations, and quality committee meetings and assigned tasks and in developing, writing, and approving protocols, policies, practice manuals, and procedures. The administrative leadership who oversee fiscal management, operations, and quality make their presence known at clinic sites to gain and share understanding of the structures, processes, and outcome measures.

The importance of communication with off-site collaborating, supervising, or specialist physicians cannot be overemphasized. Communication, be it in person, over the telephone, or by other electronic means, needs to occur among clinicians on a regular basis to promote trust in the collaborative relationships. Collaborating and supervising physicians will see patients at times, for example, if the CRNP believes the patient is beyond his or her scope of practice or is not responding to standard treatment options. Having face-to-face time with these physicians, at least quarterly if not monthly, and writing protocols and policy and practice guidelines together allows for sharing expertise. Creating referral forms with the specialty group to which the primary care practice will be referring is essential. Adding both a priority score and a specific clinical question from the CRNP can increase the likelihood of the patient's being seen and the CRNP's receiving the report back in a timely manner and with the information required. Helping CRNP clinicians to refine how they write clinical questions can be collaborative with input from the specialist.

Collaborative Teams at Work

At one NMHC that serves the chronically homeless in a major U.S. city, the NPs work with a cardiologist who comes on site once a month and sees patients at his office if a delay would have a negative impact on the patient. Several patients who were previously frequent fliers at the local emergency room (ER) have been kept out of the ER and the hospital by excellent NP and cardiologist interdisciplinary collaborative team comanagement.

Integrating on-site behavioral health services at primary care sites has allowed interdisciplinary collaborative teams to address noncompliance with medication regimes and meet self-management goals. Motivational interviewing and cognitive therapy can support patients in making incremental lifestyle changes with consistent interdisciplinary team support.

Having every member of the interdisciplinary team practice to the full extent of his or her education and training can increase quality, reduce costs, and ensure better access to care for patients; for example, the front desk staff can review records for care gaps that can be addressed during the visit or the medical assistant can ask two questions on the depression screen that will be passed to the social worker or behavioral health consultant to complete if the answers to the two questions require a more comprehensive assessment.

Diabetic educators, nutritionists, and RN care managers work together as an interdisciplinary team to teach group diabetes classes, engendering higher levels of patient engagement and group interaction and improved process and outcome measures.

COLLABORATION AND PATIENT-CENTERED MEDICAL HOMES

Collaboration and clinician-led teams are integral to the patient-centered medical home (PCMH) model, which "has gained significant momentum as a model for primary care health service reform in the U.S. as a response to the high costs and poor health-related outcomes associated with the current health care system" (Cronholm et al., 2013, p. 1).

Bleser and colleagues (2014), in studying the Pennsylvania Chronic Care Initiative, identified 13 strategies that were used to obtain practice buy-in to the PCMH model for primary care practice, with three overarching themes: effective communication, effective resource utilization, and creating a team environment. Gabbay and colleagues (2013), studying the chronic care initiative—specifically, achievement of improvement in measures related to managing and improving diabetes health indicators—found that the higher performing practices reported a stronger sense of team than did lower performing practices. There were "strong commitments to collective problem solving and shared decision making, as well as high levels of mutual trust, respect and collaboration" (Gabbay et al., 2013, p. S104). With the expectation that health care will be provided more successfully by interdisciplinary/interprofessional collaborative teams, there is a need to include more interprofessional education in formal health profession education programs.

REFERENCES

Bleser, W. K., Miller-Day, M., Naughtion, D., Bricker, P. L., Cronholm, P. F., & Gabbay, R. A. (2014). Strategies for achieving whole-practice engagement and buy-in to the patient-centered medical home. *Annals of Family Medicine, 12*(1), 37–45. doi:10.1370/afm.1564

Cronholm, P. F., Shea, J. A., Werner, R. M., Miller-Day, M., Tufano, J., Crabtree, B. F., & Gabbay, R. A. (2013). The patient centered medical home: Mental models and practice culture driving the transformation process. *Journal of General Internal Medicine, 28*(9), 1195–1201. doi:10.1007/s11606-013-2415-3

D'Amour, D., & Oandasan, I. (2004). IECPCP framework. In I. Oandasan, D. D'Amour, M. Zwarenstein, K. Barker, K. Purden, M. Beaulieau, . . . D. Treguno (Eds.), *Interdisciplinary education for collaborative, patient-centered practice: Research and findings report* (pp. 240–250). Ottawa, CAN: Health Canada. Retrieved from http://www.ferasi.umontreal.ca/eng/07_info/IECPCP_Final_Report.pdf

Drummond, N., Abbot, K., Williamson, T., & Somji, B. (2012). Interprofessional primary care in academic family medicine. *Canadian Family Physician, 58*(8), e450–e458.

Gabbay, R. A., Friedberg, M. W., Miller-Day, M., Cronholm, P. F., Adelman, A., & Schneider, E. C. (2013). A positive deviance approach to understanding key features to improving diabetes care in the medical home. *Annals of Family Medicine, 11*(1), S99–S107. doi:10.1370/afm.1473

Institute of Medicine. (2010). *The future of nursing: Leading change, advancing health.* Washington, DC: The National Academies Press.

Interprofessional Education Collaborative Expert Panel. (2011). *Core competencies for interprofessional collaborative practice: Report of an expert panel.* Washington, DC: Interprofessional Education Collaborative. Retrieved from http://www.aacn.nche.edu/education-resources/ipecreport.pdf

Somers, L. S., Marton, K. I., Barbaccia, J. C., & Randolph, J. (2000). Physician, nurse, and social worker collaboration in primary care for chronically ill seniors. *Archives of Internal Medicine, 160*(12), 1825–1833. doi:10.1001/archinte.160.12.1825

Taliani, C. A., Bricker, P. L., Adelman, A. M., Cronholm, P. F., & Gabbay, R. A. (2013). Implementing effective care management in the patient-centered medical home. *The American Journal of Managed Care, 19*(12), 957–964.

Taylor, K., Oberle, K. M., Crutcher, R. A., & Norton, P. G. (2005). Promoting health in type 2 diabetes: Nurse-physician collaboration in primary care. *Biological Research for Nursing, 6*(3), 207–215. doi:10.1177/1099800404272223

CHAPTER 6

QUALITY

Kathryn Fiandt and Nancy L. Rothman

The Institute of Medicine (IOM), as part of their landmark work on health care quality, noted that all health care should meet the following six quality standards:

- Safe—avoiding injuries to patients from the care that is intended to help them
- Effective—providing services based on scientific knowledge to all who would benefit and refraining from providing services to those not likely to benefit
- Patient centered—providing care that is respectful of and responsive to individual patient preferences, needs, and values and ensuring that patient values guide all clinical decisions
- Timely—reducing wait time and sometimes harmful delays for both those who receive treatments and those who give care
- Efficient—avoiding waste, including waste of equipment, supplies, ideas, and energy
- Equitable—providing care that does not vary in quality because of personal characteristics such as gender, ethnicity, geographic location, or socioeconomic status (Committee on Quality of Health Care in America, 2001, pp. 5–6)

Although safety is often seen as synonymous with quality, the IOM recognized that it is in fact a unique characteristic that, simply put, means that care is free of errors of both commission and omission. In 1999, in the first of several reports on health care quality, the IOM estimated that over 99,000 preventable deaths occurred annually due to health care errors. Since that report, patient safety has become a key component of all measures of health care quality; unfortunately, there is evidence that efforts to date have been ineffective. In recent testimony before the U.S. Senate, three health care experts estimated that annual preventable deaths currently range from 180,000 (Medicare population alone) to 440,000. Clearly, health care has not achieved the goal of safety as measured by the number of preventable deaths. The majority of safety deaths and errors are found in inpatient settings, and there are limited data on safety in ambulatory settings such as nurse-managed health centers (NMHCs). In ambulatory settings, because life-threatening injuries are much less common, the focus of quality improvement (QI) has been on ensuring that patients receive care that meets the other five characteristics of quality defined by the IOM. As will be apparent in the next section, although ambulatory setting quality failures do not result in lives lost as often as they do in inpatient settings, there is still a long way to go to ensure that patients receive quality care in ambulatory settings. This challenge must apply to NMHCs as well as other ambulatory settings.

QUALITY OF HEALTH CARE IN THE UNITED STATES

Although most Americans, when asked, believe that the quality of their care is the best in the world, there is ample evidence that this is not true. In a 2014 report, the Commonwealth Fund, using the previous components of quality identified by the IOM, expanded on the seven developed countries in which it regularly evaluates health care to look at a total of 11 countries, and in the update, the United States ranked at the "top" on only one measure, cost of health care per person, and this despite the fact that millions of Americans have limited access to health care or receive no care. In other words, those who receive care receive very expensive health care.

The data for the original report and the update were collected from large samples of physicians and patients. As described in Table 6.1, in the 2014 update, the United States did improve its ranking in some categories among the developed countries studied, but it continues to rank last, as it has done consistently since the 2004 report, on both health care outcomes and dimensions such as access, efficiency, and equity.

Table 6.1 Summary of the 2014 Commonwealth Fund Update

Quality: effective	Defined partially as chronic illnesses and partially as preventive medicine services	United States ranked 3 of 11
Quality: safe	Defined as mistakes reported by patients and providers	United States ranked 7 of 11
Quality: coordinated	Defined as effective communication throughout the course of treatment and across various sites	United States ranked 6 of 11
Quality: patient centered	Defined as care delivered with the patients' needs and preferences in mind	United States ranked 4 of 11
Accessible	Defined by affordability and access to timely attention	Affordable: United States ranked 11 of 11 Timeliness: United States ranked 5 of 11
Efficient	Defined as national per capita costs, but also includes indicators such as excess paperwork hassle and using the ER when primary care is available	United States ranked 11 of 11
Equitable	Defined as care that does not vary in quality due to personal characteristics like race or gender	United States ranked 11 of 11
Healthy lives	Defined as preventable deaths, infant mortality, and healthy life expectancy (at age 60)	United States ranked 11 of 11*

*It is relevant to note how much worse the United States performed on these markers. There were 96 preventable deaths per 100,000 in the United States, followed by the United Kingdom at 83/100,000; France had the fewest, only 55/100,000. For infant mortality, the United States had 6.1 deaths per 1,000 live births; the next highest was New Zealand with 5.5, and Sweden had the fewest, 2.3/1,000. Healthy life expectancy at age 60 in the United States was 17.5 years; only Norway ranked lower, with 17.4 years, and Switzerland ranked the highest at 19 years.

ER, Emergency room.

Source: Davis, Stremikis, Squires, & Schoen (2014).

The conclusion of the 2014 update is that in the United States, if health care is received, it is generally safe, appropriate, coordinated, and patient centered compared with other countries, but that U.S. health care is inefficient. This inefficiency results in increased resource (time and money) use for both providers and patients; significant variability in access to care and in quality of care received; and, despite the high costs, poor outcomes as measured by preventable deaths, infant mortality, and healthy life expectancy.

In the report, the authors discuss the impact of the Affordable Care Act (ACA). As they noted, while insurance will undoubtedly improve access, even insured people in the United States reported less stability in their care and higher out-of-pocket expenses, both of which negatively impact health. In other words, insurance is important, but not sufficient for improving overall health.

The Commonwealth Fund is not the only large organization to evaluate the quality of health care in the United States. The Agency for Healthcare Research and Quality (AHRQ) prepares annual reports on both quality and disparities using similar criteria (2013a and 2013b), and their findings are similar to those of the Commonwealth Fund. AHRQ's disparities report (2013a), which addresses problems among the populations that often seek service at NMHCs, continues to indicate that both being a racial or ethnic minority and living in poverty have a significant negative impact on the quality of care received.

Quality and NMHCs

Health care delivered in NMHCs should, at a minimum, be safe, although quality is the key standard for ambulatory care. This means that care is not only safe, but, as noted by the IOM, evidence based, cost effective, accessible, equable, and patient centered. This also means avoiding waste, measured as misuse (e.g., prescribing unnecessary antibiotics), overuse of resources (e.g., ordering unnecessary diagnostic tests), and resource underuse (e.g., failure to order or perform recommended screening tests).

As noted earlier, there is less evidence for safety problems in ambulatory settings and more data regarding quality, and there are limited data that compare NMHCs with other ambulatory practices on quality measures. However, a significant body of literature describes the quality and outcomes of NMHC practices, and this literature is reviewed in this chapter.

NMHCs are a small portion of the ambulatory practice community in the United States, and, as might be expected, there are fewer data regarding the quality of NMHC care. However, over the years there have been multiple wide-ranging reports that conclude that the health care provided by nurse practitioners (NPs) is consistently equivalent to physician care, that it is safe and appropriate, and that patients are highly satisfied (Brown & Grimes, 1995; Laurant et al., 2005; Office of Technological Assessment, 1986). Most recently, a large multidisciplinary team conducted a comprehensive review of the literature (Stanik-Hutt et al., 2013). The authors reviewed 37 studies and used 11 outcomes classified as quality, safety, or effectiveness. They, too, found no difference or slightly better outcomes in all areas when comparing NP care with that provided by physicians.

To date, all studies have supported the conclusion that NP care is at minimum as safe as that provided by physicians and occasionally results in greater patient satisfaction. A subset of the literature, however, studies quality in NMHCs and often looks beyond safety and satisfaction to other measures of quality. In this section, the literature regarding quality in nurse-managed centers is reviewed and differentiated from other QI studies.

Comparison of NMHCs With National Data Sets

The Uniform Data System

One major study (Pohl, Tanner, Pilon, & Benkert, 2011) compared 4 years of national nursing center data with data from federally qualified health centers (FQHCs) using FQHC Uniform Data System (UDS) data and available overlapping data. It was determined that both FQHCs and NMHCs served diverse patient populations. The more significant variation was regarding the sources of revenue. In FQHCs, 60% of practice revenue came from patient care, whereas at NMHCs, patient care accounted for only 40% of revenue. Both practice types relied heavily on grants, but NMHCs relied much more heavily on donations and subsidies, primarily university support. This dependence on university support has been a consistent weakness in NMHC practices because schools cannot always keep up the support.

Another significant finding was that FQHCs actually had fewer uninsured patients but received cost-based reimbursement for all patients. NMHCs had fewer insured patients, and when they did receive Medicaid payments, they were often at lower rates. The presence of more uninsured patients is supported by another study (Fiandt, Doeschot, Lanning, & Latkze, 2010) that characterized NMHC patients as more "vulnerable" than the patients at federally subsidized practices. In this study, more NMHC patients were more likely to report being uninsured, not having primary care providers, and not having received care in the past year due to cost than were patients of urban Indian FHQCs or rural health clinics. They also reported higher percentages of hypertension, diabetes, and depression than did the other patients.

Health Plan Employer Data and Information Set

Two studies have compared the performance of NMHC practices with the Health Plan Employer Data and Information Set (HEDIS) of the National Committee for Quality Assurance (NCQA) data. Barkauskas, Pohl, Benkert, and Wells (2005) used HEDIS to evaluate the quality of practice at six NMHCs in the Michigan Academic Consortium. All NMHCs served a vulnerable population, and all centers exceeded the HEDIS 50th percentile standard with a focus on chronic health problems, specifically asthma, cervical cancer screening, diabetes, and hypertension management. In two areas, smoking cessation and mammography, NMHCs did not meet the 50th percentile, which the authors attributed to difficulty in obtaining the data (e.g., the mammogram was ordered, but it was difficult to receive reports from outside agencies, or patients were unable to obtain due to costs). Coddington, Sands, Edwards, Kirkpatrick, and Chen (2011) used HEDIS metrics to evaluate the care received at an NMHC that provided pediatric care. This study focused on childhood immunizations, upper respiratory infections, and access to primary care providers. In this practice, the clinicians met or exceeded all of the HEDIS measures. It is of note that both NMHC practices provided care to vulnerable patients at risk for poor outcomes due to poverty, lack of insurance, and/or demographic risks such as minority status.

Quality Studies Conducted at NMHCs

Two sets of articles describe comprehensive NMHC QI programs: the early work of the Northern Illinois University and the work of the Michigan Academic Consortium, in partnership with the Institute for Nursing Centers.

Anderko and her colleagues at Northern Illinois University published several articles reporting on 5 years of QI data at their NMHC in rural Illinois (Anderko, Uscian, & Robertson, 1999). Like other NMHCs, they reported improvement in chronic health problems and patient satisfaction (Anderko & Uscian, 2001) and reported good-to-excellent clinical outcomes.

In addition to these traditional reports, Anderko and her team added two critical additional components to their practice evaluation and improvement. First, they introduced an expanded conceptual definition of access (Anderko, Robertson, & Uscian, 2000) using Penchansky and Thomas's model (1981), which identifies five subcategories: *availability* (i.e., number and type of services and resources in relation to the patients' needs); *accessibility* (i.e., the location of the facility and its clients, the distance, available transportation, travel time, and costs); *accommodation* (i.e., how resources are organized to accept clients, including hours of operation, phone access, walk-in availability, bilingual services, etc.); *adaptability* (i.e., the patients' perception of the providers' personal characteristics and the health care facility's physical characteristics); and *affordability* (i.e., costs in relation to patients' ability to pay).

Subsequently, Anderko and her team reported on job satisfaction among NMHC employees (Anderko, Robertson, & Lewis, 1999) and students' satisfaction with their clinical experiences at the centers (Robertson, Anderko, & Uscian, 2000). These three added metrics (expanded access, job satisfaction, and student satisfaction) should be included in all NMHC quality programs.

More recently, Pohl and the Michigan Academic Consortium have published extensively in the area of QI in NMHCs. In addition to the HEDIS study described in the previous section, work has been published on patient satisfaction (Benkert, Barkauskas, Pohl, Tanner, & Nagelkirk, 2002). This study of 907 patients at seven NMHCs used a standard satisfaction tool.

Additional literature focuses on individual interventions or outcomes, and several articles have described patient satisfaction. In addition, Bryant and Graham (2002) reported very high patient satisfaction in a sample of 506 of their NMHCs, and Cole, Mackey, and Lindenberg (2001) reported on a small study that evaluated the impact of wait times on patient satisfaction.

Clinical outcomes have been the focus of other studies. Benkert, Buchholz, and Poole (2001) reported improved control and no difference in the clinical outcomes of African American men with hypertension between those with and without insurance. Mackey, Cole, and Lindenberg (2005), in a small study of patients with type 2 diabetes, found significant improvement in care processes, but none in clinical outcomes. This is a common finding, and this study attributed the finding to the short time between implementing and measuring the outcomes. Additionally, this study provides a nice summary of the process for implementing QI across the care continuum. Dontje and Forrest (2011) recently published a useful description of the impact of group visits on the health status and satisfaction of patients with type 2 diabetes; a central conclusion was that there was a dose effect and that for measurable improvement, patients had to participate in at least three such visits. All of these are QI studies that can have a significant impact on future health care. With more Doctor of Nursing Practice students doing QI projects, ideally in NMHCs, we anticipate a higher number of NPs with strong QI skills and more literature that describes the impact of practice interventions on health outcomes.

Cost Data

The Michigan Academic Consortium, under the leadership of Pohl, has been committed to capturing fiscal data on NMHC practices, which have traditionally resisted addressing real-world costs and thus becoming competitive. Coddington and Sands (2008), in a review of literature on costs and outcomes, reported that the data were weak. Some of their studies compared NMHC costs with those for emergency department (ED) visits and patient satisfaction, while others looked at expenses compared with physicians' costs. Often the practices, given the socially complex needs of the patients and the NP model, actually reported higher costs than did traditional medical practices. All researchers studying NMHC costs say that more systematic cost and outcomes data are needed to justify reimbursement at levels that cover costs and that NMHCs should be more open to increasing volume.

Standardized Data Sets

Since the advent of NMHCs, there has been pressure to develop a standard set of data that all clinics can use to describe their practices, patients, clinical outcomes, and other information. The goal is twofold: to ensure that NMHCs are capturing data that will allow them to compare outcomes with more traditional medical practices and to capture the practice characteristics that might differentiate the NMHC from traditional medical practices. Previous descriptions of studies comparing NMHC data against the UDS and HEDIS data sets are excellent examples of ensuring that NMHCs are benchmarked against health care system standards. However, there is also research aimed at capturing the differences with NMHCs. Barton, Baramee, Sowers, and Robertson (2003) referred to NMHC care as "value-added," while Fiandt, Laux, Sarver, and Sayer (2002) referred to "finding the nurse in NP practice." Both Fiandt and her colleagues and Haugsdal and Scherb (2003) used nursing intervention classifications to describe NP practices, while Barton and her team used the Omaha model. Both of these frameworks have been used successfully to capture aspects of NMHC practice that might not be found using traditional Current Procedural Terminology (CPT) and International Classification of Diseases (ICD)-9/10 codes.

Conclusion of the NMHC QI Literature Review

Although the literature is scant, it is clear that when compared with other quality projects, NMHCs have good outcomes and high patient satisfaction. In addition, authors have looked at other quality metrics, including costs, an expanded definition of access, employee and student satisfaction, and social determinants of health. These additional metrics should become the norm as an increasing number of Doctor of Nursing Practice students and graduates begin conducting QI projects, ideally in nurse-managed practices and with an expanded definition of quality.

QUALITY PROCESSES

Having reviewed the nature of quality in ambulatory settings, evidence of poor quality outcomes in the U.S. health system, and the literature on QI in NMHCs, we now briefly review the process for conducting QI evaluations and then review national programs that encourage QI.

Key components:

- *Data.* Whether in the form of a paper or electronic health records, data that ensure quality depend on the ability to measure the components for evidence at baseline and over time.
- *Interprofessional teams.* Quality in any setting is not the role or responsibility of any one person. The evaluation and improvement of care require that the entire team be committed to data collection and improvement.
- *Organizational support.* Quality cannot be accomplished without the support from practice leadership. This means a commitment to fiscal resources, time for improvement projects, and improvement processes.

Key Questions Regarding QI

- What is the aim of the QI process in a particular situation? At one point in time in any practice, QI may be focused on decreasing the no-show rate, while at a different time or practice, the goal might be to improve outcomes for patients with type 2 diabetes. Individual centers will need to assess their needs on an ongoing basis.
- How will we know if the changes we make are an improvement? This starts with baseline data that address the question, "How do we know we have a problem?" The next step is to ask, "What are the standards of care for this issue?" For example, a practice may find that its patients with type 2 diabetes have an average A1c of 8, and the standard ranges from 7 to 7.5 based on national guidelines. With no-shows, the practice might find that its rates are well below the national average; therefore, although no-shows disrupt practice, it may not be worth the time and effort to improve the rate.
- What changes can be made in the practice that will result in improvement? Evidence-based practice comes into play as NMHCs explore interventions that have worked in other practices and might be feasible. Other sources of intervention models are collaboratives or similar practices that are willing to share successful strategies.

Quality Metrics

The Commonwealth Fund report reviewed earlier is an excellent example of a variety of metrics and data sources that are used to measure quality. The Institute for Healthcare Improvement identifies three categories of measures that should be considered in QI: outcomes, process, and balancing. Outcomes are the traditional patient-centered measures, comprising physical measures like blood pressure and A1c, but also patient quality of life and functional status. Process measures address what the health care team "does" and include things like returning phone calls, performing annual foot checks, and ensuring that the primary care provider receives copies of reports. Balancing measures are measures of how well the system is working and include items like patient satisfaction and no-show rates.

Many sources of metrics and benchmarks or standards are available for nurse-managed practices. Some are disease based, for example, the American Diabetic Association Standard for Practice; some are system based, for example, The Joint Commission Primary Care Medical Home; and some are developed by professional organizations. NMHC-specific metrics were discussed in the previous section, and the National Nursing Centers Consortium's (NNCC's) "Quality Standards for Nurse Managed Health Clinics" (www.nncc.us/site/pdf/NMHC_Quality_Standards.pdf) is reviewed in the next section.

Accountability for Quality

There is great pressure in the U.S. health care system to improve quality. Federal efforts by the Centers for Medicaid and Medicare have funded practices to expand information system capacity through the meaningful use component of the ACA, which also ties reimbursement to "value"-based care, increasing reimbursement for high quality and lowering it for low quality.

For over 15 years, national organizations have been building databases of quality metrics that are now being used to measure value in federal value-based reimbursement programs. And since 2007, the medical community has established standards for what are termed patient-centered medical homes (PCMHs; NCQA, www.ncqa.org/Programs/Recognition/Practices/PatientCenteredMedicalHomePCMH.aspx) or primary care medical homes (The Joint Commission). Both The Joint Commission and NCQA have processes for accrediting PCMHs, and several NMHCs have achieved PCMH accreditation. The best description of PCMHs and related metrics was published in 2010 (Strange et al., 2010) in the *Journal of General Internal Medicine*. Although the article is clearly physician centric, the reader will find an excellent review of the concept and of metrics that build on the original IOM definition of primary care (Donaldson, Yordy, Lohr, & Vanselow, 1996). A key component of accreditation for all forms of health care delivery is a viable QI program; this is referred to in the article but not elaborated on. Two other key concepts that are missing are team-based care and population health. Most recently, it has been more clearly recognized that primary care and health care homes require highly functional teams and need data in order to see patients not just as individuals and families but as a population and to support system-level improvement as described in the QI section of this chapter.

THE NATIONAL NURSING CENTER NMHC CERTIFICATION INITIATIVE

In 2014, the NNCC announced an NMHC certification process based on NNCC standards. This certification is designed to serve multiple functions:

- For NMHCs *with PCMH certification*, this certification clarifies the distinct differences between an NMHC and a traditional practice. A dually certified practice extends beyond the PCMH to include the value-added components of the NMHC certification standards.
- For *established NMHCs that have not begun a certification process*, the self-study required for initial NMHC certification would be an ideal first step for reviewing where the practice is and what they need to improve as they move forward.
- For *NMHCs in the early stages of practice*, the NNCC standards serve as benchmarks for the key components that should be reflected in their practices. These standards can be integrated into business plans and grant applications to emphasize the applying practice's attention to quality and national standards.
- For *people considering developing NMHCs*, the quality and safety guidelines should serve as a basic checklist of all of the aspects of practice development that need to be taken into account. They provide guides for leadership to clarify the necessary time, funding, and personnel commitments for establishing a successful NMHC.

The NMHC certification process consists of reviewing all NMHC guidelines. Practice leadership is asked to attest to the degree to which the practice has met each standard (met, partially met, not met, and not applicable). A list of documents that support the attestations is required, and responses of not applicable or partially met require clarification and justification. Table 6.2 provides a more detailed comparison of NNCC's certification standards compared with those of both NCQA and The Joint Commission.

Table 6.2 Comparison of NMHC Quality and Safety Standards With Joint Commission Primary Care Home (2011 Working Draft) and NCQA Patient-Centered Medical Home (2011 Working Draft)

NMHC STANDARDS	JOINT COMMISSION	NCQA
Mission	Definition	Six Standards/Goals

• Increase access
• Eliminate health disparities
• Definition of primary care—care is comprehensive, coordinated, and continuous for acute and chronic health problems and a wide range of health promotion activities
	• A medical home is a primary care model that has the following core functions and attributes:
	  ■ Comprehensive, coordinated, patient-centered care
	  ■ Superb access to care
	  ■ A systems-based approach to quality and safety
		• Ensure accessibility and continuity
		• Identify and manage patient populations
		• Plan and manage care
		• Provide self-management support
		• Track and coordinate care
		• Utilize performance measures and QI evaluation
		
		Goal: to make it feasible for primary care practices to move toward improved quality, reduced waste, and an enhanced patient experience

Nursing Model	Patient Centeredness	Patient Centeredness/Increased Emphasis on Patient Feedback
The clinic reflects a nursing model that includes • Patient centeredness • Primary, secondary, and tertiary prevention • Community orientation, including partnering with community agencies • Patient education and nurse case management as core components of service • Support of education of health professionals	• Each patient has a patient-selected PCC • The PCC and the interdisciplinary team work in partnership with the patient • Each patient's culture, language, and education needs are considered • Patient is involved in establishing treatment plan • Support for patient self-management is provided • The organization provides patient education and training based on needs; health literacy is taken into consideration • The organization respects the patient's rights regarding treatment received, information, and participation in decisions	• Enable continuity of care with same provider • Provide access to care after hours • Expand survey categories to include items such as access, communication, coordination, comprehension, shared decision making, and whole-person orientation • Use survey data for QI • Involve patients and families in QI

Quality and Safety	Systems-Based Approach to Quality and Safety	Performance Measures and QI
• Formal QI program is benchmarked with national standards • Emergency plans are in place • Clinic meets national standards and legal and regulatory requirements • Practice is evidence based • Patient satisfaction is monitored and is taken into consideration for QI	• Use evidence-based practice • Use clinical decision support tools • Use electronic health information technology • Provide care to a "panel" of patients	• Requires increased number of performance measures • Requires monitoring for utilization and overuse data • Requires practice to demonstrate improvement

Outcomes	Systems-Based Approach to Quality and Safety	Align Processes to Improve Quality and Reduce Waste
• Heath record, preferably electronic, is in place to perform patient registry functions as well as to monitor individual patients • Data are collected that reflect care processes, clinical outcomes, and balancing outcomes • Data are collected that reflect the impact of the clinic on health disparities and increased access to care • When appropriate, data collection is IRB approved	• Measures patients' responses to care and satisfaction • Practices population health management • Involves patient in performance measures • Compiles and analyzes data in usable formats; compares internal data over time and compares with external data; all data comparisons are used for QI • The organization improves performance	• Use electronic health record • Practice e-prescribing • Track unscheduled hospitalizations and ER visits • Have regular reconciliation of medications

(continued)

Table 6.2 Comparison of NMHC Quality and Safety Standards With Joint Commission Primary Care Home (2011 Working Draft) and NCQA Patient-Centered Medical Home (2011 Working Draft) (*continued*)

NMHC STANDARDS	JOINT COMMISSION	NCQA
Primary Care/Coordination	**Comprehensive Care**	**Coordination of Care**
• Services include facilitating access to the health care system	• Care includes acute, preventive, and chronic illness and disease management	• Coordinate referrals or other providers and community service agencies
• Health needs and problems are addressed at the individual, family, and community levels • Practice reflects interprofessional collaboration • Care is culturally appropriate	• Care is continuous, comprehensive, and across the life span • A team-based approach is used • Internal and external resources are identified to meet patients' needs • The PCC has the education and skills to handle most patients' health care problems	• Arrange for information exchange between facilities including after-hours care
Access to Care	**Superb Access to Care**	**Access and Continuity**
• Services include access to specialists • The clinic increases access to people who are at risk for health disparities • Services are available at times and locations that meet the needs of patients and the community • Services are acceptable to the patients being served • Services are affordable	• Available 24 hours a day, 7 days a week • Access for non-visit-related patient needs • Access for patients with special communication needs • Use of electronic media and flexible appointment scheduling • Shorter wait times for appointments, especially in response to acute problems	• Access to care during and after hours

Sustainability | **Not Addressed**

- The budget is sufficient to maintain the practice
- The budget reflects and supports the mission and strategic plan

Practice Leadership | **Systems-Based Approach to Quality and Safety**

- The clinic leadership supports the nursing model
- Strategic and business plans are in place that serve as the basis for major decisions
- Policies and procedures are in place to ensure that operations are standardized
- The clinic has an advisory board that includes consumers/patients and staff
- Employee satisfaction is regularly evaluated
- The work environment is considered safe and supportive of all employees; all employees feel their voice is heard

- The PCC and team members function within their scope of practice
- The PCC and team members practice in accordance with regulations, including privileges granted as well as other laws
- Leaders establish priorities for performance improvement
- Organization leadership communicates priority of safety to all personnel, patients and families, and interested external parties

Physical Environment | **Not Addressed**

- Meets ADA and OSHA standards
- Hazardous waste policies are in place

(continued)

Table 6.2 Comparison of NMHC Quality and Safety Standards With Joint Commission Primary Care Home (2011 Working Draft) and NCQA Patient–Centered Medical Home (2011 Working Draft) (*continued*)

NMHC STANDARDS	JOINT COMMISSION	NCQA
Not Present but Implied in Nursing Model	**Behavioral Health**	**Integrate Behaviors Affecting Health, Mental Health, and Substance Abuse**
• The clinic addresses the needs of the whole patient to include biopsychosocial-spiritual concerns as they impact the patient's health and well-being • Behavioral and mental health issues are addressed as part of the management of all health problems	• Behavioral health needs are included under "access to care, treatment, and services"	• Comprehensive mental health assessments • One of three "clinically important conditions" identified must relate to an unhealthy behavior or substance abuse or mental health problems • Track referrals and coordination of care for mental health and substance abuse

ADA, Americans with Disabilities Act; ER, emergency room; NCQA, National Committee for Quality Assurance; NMHC, nurse-managed health center; OSHA, Occupational Safety & Health Administration; PCC, primary care clinician; QI, quality improvement.

A CASE STUDY

We conclude this chapter with a case study of one NMHC and its work with both QI and PCMH accreditation, the Pennsylvania Chronic Care Initiative (PACCI).

"In 2007, government and health care leaders in Pennsylvania were reaching a growing consensus that some form of action must be taken to address the state's alarming and growing, chronic disease burden" (History of Pennsylvania's Chronic Care Initiative, 2012). AHRQ reported that Pennsylvania's chronic illness hospital admission rates were three times the national average. Asthma admission rates were three times the rates for the best-performing states, and diabetes admission rates were four times higher. The governor appointed a 45-member commission made up of providers, payers, hospitals, health systems, businesses, labor, consumers, and state agency representatives. The 2008 Pennsylvania Chronic Care Management, Reimbursement and Cost Reduction Commission's strategic plan identified a goal:

> To improve care and reduce health care costs, we must transform chronic care treatment in the Commonwealth, beginning with the nature and structure of primary care delivery, continuing with the provision of self-management support for patients with one or more chronic diseases and culminating with the alignment of incentives that motivate primary care teams and patients to improve the management of chronic illness.

The commission elected to use Ed Wagner's Chronic Care Model and its rapid cycle testing for practice improvements and elements of PCMHs, and it required practices to receive NCQA PCMH recognition within 12 to 18 months in order to continue participating in the initiative. Four strategies were implemented (History of Pennsylvania's Chronic Care Initiative, 2012):

1. A new primary care reimbursement model that used the Chronic Care Model, practice team collaboration, care coordination, evidence-based practice, assistance to patients in setting and achieving self-management goals, and linguistically and culturally competent care
2. Holding regional learning collaboratives based on the Chronic Care Model
3. Requiring monthly reporting on process and clinical outcome measures from participating practices
4. Creating high-risk registries and hiring registered nurses to provide practice-based care management

The PACCI began in the southeast corner of Pennsylvania, in Philadelphia, Montgomery, Chester, Delaware, and Bucks counties. Eight nurse-led primary care clinics, all NNCC members, were selected to participate, and all obtained NCQA recognition as PCMHs. *History of Pennsylvania's Chronic Care Initiative* (2012) reports that diabetes measures for July 2008 to January 2012, including HbA1C > 9 reduced by 14%; blood pressure < 140/90 improved by 16%; self-management goal setting improved by 37%; and foot exams increased by 41%.

A RAND study on the PACCI (Friedberg, Schneider, Rosenthal, Volpp, & Werner, 2014), which is described as "one of the earliest and largest multipayer medical home pilots conducted in the United States," reported limited improvements in quality and no association with reduced hospital, emergency room, ambulatory, or total costs over 3 years. Practices that participated in a 2013 PACCI learning collaborative indicated that primary care has little control over hospital or specialty practice resource use and that they needed additional time to measure the initiative's impact.

Independence Blue Cross of Philadelphia recently announced, "Results from a three-year study [2009 to 2011] involving 700 of its high-risk members show those cared for in patient-centered medical homes experienced reduced costs and service utilization, when compared to other patients" (George, 2014, p. 1). Although more time is needed to evaluate such multipayer projects, it is marvelous to see the inclusion of NMHCs in these important initiatives that can lead to improved care and reduced health care costs.

CONCLUSION

NMHCs have an opportunity to become integral components of the expanding primary health care delivery system in the United States. NMHC practices provide safe, quality health care delivered by NPs and other health care team members. Research suggests that their patients are highly satisfied, that the clinics serve patients who would often go without care or who are vulnerable to poor outcomes or disparities, and that the clinicians are trusted by their patients. These are critical components of a successful primary care practice.

However, because of the small number of NMHCs compared with traditional medical practices, and due to the limited fiscal support, NMHCs have produced limited data on clinical outcomes, and there is insufficient evidence that the practices incorporate rigorous QI programs. Additionally, it is still difficult to differentiate NMHCs from traditional medical practices.

NNCC's NMHC quality standard resources, and now the opportunity for NMHC certification, are critical steps in demonstrating the value of the services provided by NMHCs at levels that describe for policy makers and insurers the impact of care, differentiated practice, and cost savings. A national movement of NMHCs' adopting these standards, obtaining certification, and moving into the mainstream of practice improvement at the national level will ensure that NMHCs receive the recognition they are due and have the opportunity to be essential providers in the evolving U.S. health care system.

REFERENCES

Agency for Healthcare Research and Quality (AHRQ). (2013a). *2012 National healthcare disparities report.* Rockville, MD. Retrieved from http://www.ahrq.gov/research/findings/nhqrdr/nhdr12/

Agency for Healthcare Research and Quality (AHRQ). (2013b). *2012 National healthcare quality report.* Rockville, MD. Retrieved from http://www.ahrq.gov/research/findings/nhqrdr/nhqr12/

Anderko, L., Robertson, J. F., & Lewis, P. (1999). Job satisfaction in a rural differentiated practice setting. *Nursing Connections, 12*(1), 49–58.

Anderko, L., Robertson, J. F., & Uscian, M. M. (2000). The effectiveness of a rural nursing center in improving health access in a three-county area. *The Journal of Rural Health, 16*(2), 177–184. doi:10.1111/j.1748-0361.2000.tb00452.x

Anderko, L., & Uscian, M. M. (2001). Quality outcome measures at an academic rural nurse-managed center: A core safety net provider. *Policy, Politics, & Nursing Practice, 2*(4), 288–294. doi:10.1177/152715440100200406

Anderko, L., Uscian, M. M., & Robertson, J. F. (1999). Improving client outcomes through a differentiated practice: A rural nursing center model. *Public Health Nursing, 16*(3), 168–175.

Barkauskas, V., Pohl, J., Benkert, R., & Wells, M. (2005). Measuring quality in nurse-managed centers using HEDIS measures. *Journal of Healthcare Quality, 27*(1), 4–14. doi:10.1111/j.1945-1474.2005.tb00540.x

Barton, A., Baramee, J., Sowers, D., & Robertson, K. (2003). Articulating the value-added dimension of NP care. *The Nurse Practitioner, 28*(12), 34–40.

Benkert, R., Barkauskas, V., Pohl, J., Tanner, C., & Nagelkirk, J. (2002). Patient satisfaction outcomes in nurse-managed centers. *Outcomes Management, 6*(4), 174–177.

Benkert, R., Buchholz, S., & Poole, M. (2001). Hypertension outcomes in an urban nurse-managed center. *Journal of the American Academy of Nurse Practitioners, 13*(2), 84–89. doi: 10.1111/j.1745-7599.2001.tb00223.x

Brown, S., & Grimes, D. (1995). A meta-analysis of nurse practitioners and nurse midwives in primary care. *Nursing Research, 44*(6), 332–339.

Bryant, R., & Graham, M. (2002). Advanced practice nurses: A study of client satisfaction. *Journal of the American Academy of Nurse Practitioners, 14*(2), 88–92. doi:10.1111/j.1745-7599.2002.tb00096.x

Coddington, J., & Sands, L. (2008). Cost of health care and quality outcomes of patients at nurse-managed clinics. *Nursing Economics, 26*(2), 75–84.

Coddington, J., Sands, L., Edwards, N., Kirkpatrick, J., & Chen, S. (2011). Quality of health care provided at a pediatric nurse-managed clinic. *Journal of the American Academy of Nurse Practitioners, 23*(12), 674-680. doi: 10.1111/j.1745-7599.2011 .00657.x

Cole, F., Mackey, T., & Lindenberg, J. (2001). Wait time and satisfaction with care and service at a nurse practitioner managed clinic. *Journal of the American Academy of Nurse Practitioners, 13*(10), 467–472. doi:10.1111/j.1745-7599.2001.tb00008.x

Committee on Quality of Health Care in America. (2001). *Crossing the quality chasm: A new health system for the 21st century.* Washington, DC: National Academies Press.

Davis, K., Stremikis, K., Squires, D., & Schoen, C. (2014). *Mirror, mirror on the wall: How the performance of the U.S. health care system compares internationally.* New York, NY: The Commonwealth Fund.

Donaldson, M. S., Yordy, K. D., Lohr, K. N., & Vanselow, N. A. (Eds.). (1996). *Primary care: America's health in a new era.* Washington, DC: National Academies Press.

Dontje, K., & Forrest, K. (2011). Implementing group visits: Are they effective in improving diabetes self-management outcomes? *The Journal for Nurse Practitioners, 7*(7), 571–577. doi:10.1016/j.nurpra.2010.09.014

Fiandt, K., Doeschot, C., Lanning, J., & Latzke, L. (2010). Characteristics of risk in patients of nurse practitioner safety net practices. *Journal of the American Academy of Nurse Practitioners, 22*(9), 474–479. doi:10.1111/j.1745-7599.2010.00536.x

Fiandt, K., Laux, C., Sarver, N., & Sayer, R. J. (2002). Finding the nurse in nurse practitioner practice: A pilot study of rural family nurse practitioner practice. *Clinical Excellence for Nurse Practitioners, 5*(6), 13–21.

Friedberg, M. W., Schneider, E. C., Rosenthal, M. B., Volpp, K. G., & Werner, R. M. (2014). Association between participation in a multipayer medical home intervention and changes in quality, utilization and costs of care. *Journal of the American Medical Association, 311*(8), 815–825. doi:10.1001/jama.2014.353

George, J. (2014, March 24). Independence Blue Cross says medical homes helping high-risk members [Web log comment]. *Philadelphia Business Journal.* Retrieved from http://www.bizjournals.com/philadelphia/blog/health-care/2014/03/ independence-blue-cross-says-medical-homes-helping.html?page=all

Haugsdal, C., & Scherb, C. (2003). Using nursing interventions classification to describe the work of the nurse practitioner. *Journal of the American Academy of Nurse Practitioners, 15*(2), 87–94.

History of Pennsylvania's Chronic Care Initiative. (2012). Retrieved from http:// paspreaddotcom.files.wordpress.com/2012/02/pa-cci-history-final.pdf

Laurant, M., Reeves, D., Hermens, R., Braspenning, J., Grol, R., & Sibbald, B. (2005 April 18). Substitution of doctors by nurses in primary care. *Cochrane Database Syst Rev.* 2005:CD001271.

Mackey, T., Cole, F., & Lindenberg, J. (2005). Quality improvement and changes in diabetic patient outcomes in an academic nurse practitioner primary care practice. *Journal of the American Academy of Nurse Practitioners, 17*(12), 547–553.

Office of Technology Assessment. (1986). *Nurse practitioners, physician assistants, and certified nurse midwives: A policy analysis.* Washington, DC: US Government Printing Office.

Penchansky, R., & Thomas, J. W. (1981). The concept of access: Definition and relationship to consumer satisfaction. *Medical Care, 19*(2), 127–140. doi: 10.1097/00005650 -198102000-00001

Pohl, J. M., Tanner, C., Pilon, B., & Benkert, R. (2011). Comparison of nurse managed health centers with community health centers as safety net providers. *Policy, Politics, & Nursing Practice, 12*(2) 90–99. doi: 10.1177/1527154411417882

Robertson, J. F., Anderko, L., & Uscian, M. M. (2000). Nursing students' evaluation of clinical experience in a rural differentiated-practice setting. *Nursing Connections, 13*(1), 43–52.

Stanik-Hutt, J., Newhouse, R., White, K., Johantgen, M., Bass, E., Zangaro, G., . . . Weiner, J. (2013). The quality and effectiveness of care provided by nurse practitioners. *The Journal for Nurse Practitioners, 9*(8), 492–500. doi:10.1016/j. nurpra.2013.07.004

Strange, K., Nutting, P., Miller, W., Jaen, C., Crabtree, B., Flocke, S., & Gill, J. (2010). Defining and measuring the patient-centered medical home. *Journal of General Internal Medicine, 25*(6), 601–612. doi:10.1007/s11606-010-1291-3

Patient Satisfaction With Care Received in Nurse-Managed Primary Care Clinics: The Numbers and the Stories

Eunice S. King and Nancy L. Rothman

As a newer model of primary care delivery, nurse-managed health care clinics (NMHCs) are concerned about monitoring their patients' experience and satisfaction with the care received. A retrospective observational study of a random sample of 41,209 patient satisfaction surveys provided by adult and pediatric medicine departments from 1997 to 2000 (Roblin, Becker, Adams, Howard, & Roberts, 2004, p. 579) reported that patients were "significantly more likely to be satisfied with practitioner interaction on visits attended by physician assistants/nurse practitioners than visits attended by MDs." Satisfaction with access to care or overall experience did not differ by type of clinician. A study by Michael, Schaffer, Egan, Little, and Pritchard (2013, p. 50) found "a strong and inverse relationship between patient satisfaction and wait times in ambulatory care settings," underscoring the importance of measuring many aspects of the patient experience because doing so "can be an important strategy for transforming practices" (Browne, Roseman, Shaller, & Edgman-Levitan, 2010, p. 921).

This chapter reports on the satisfaction of patients receiving care in one of five nurse-managed health centers that comprise an NMHC network in Philadelphia. Collectively, these centers serve roughly 11,200 patients annually, some of whom are homeless and many of whom are public housing residents. Each of the clinics is located in an urban area and is a safety net provider for traditionally underserved, minority populations, who typically suffer from health disparities.

Each year in April, a paper-and-pencil survey is distributed to the first 100 clients receiving care in each of the clinics. After their visit with the health care provider, patients are asked to complete a 1-page, 14-item questionnaire that was adapted from the Medical Outcomes Trust Patient Satisfaction survey, which is no longer available. Aspects of the care assessed by this instrument are (a) length of time to obtain an appointment; (b) convenience of the clinic location; (c) ease of phone access to the clinic; (d) appointment wait times; (e) amount of time the clinician spent with the patient; (f) explanation of what was done for the patient; (g) clinical staff's technical skills (thoroughness, carefulness, and competence); (h) clinic staff's personal manner (courtesy, respect, sensitivity, and friendliness); (i) maintenance of confidentiality of information; (j) information provided to improve health; (k) patients' confidence in their ability to manage their health problems; and (l) likelihood of recommending the health center to family and friends.

When the survey has been completed by 100 patients in each network clinic, the data are reviewed by the quality improvement or quality assurance committee and used to guide practice transformation. Results of the patient satisfaction survey have enabled this network to recognize (a) when extended wait times for appointments required expanded physical space with additional exam rooms and clinical staff and (b) when getting through to the office by phone was taking too long, necessitating the establishment of a call center. In addition, comments in the free response section by the homeless patients suggested that a clinic needed to be open at 7 a.m., as opposed to staying open late, to meet the needs of homeless patients in shelters, who are frequently asked to leave shelters early in the morning but need to be back by 6 p.m. to get a bed for the night.

Table 7.1 shows the aggregated results of the patient satisfaction survey conducted by the five network centers in April 2013. As in prior years, the individual item scores are relatively high, the relatively lower scores being for the length of time the patient waited for an appointment, the length of time waiting at the office to be seen, and getting through to the office by telephone. In addition to the annual paper-and-pencil survey, in 2014 the network conducted a focus group to provide patients with an opportunity to voice their satisfaction and/or dissatisfaction with the clinic and the care they received. In relying solely on quantitative data from the satisfaction

Table 7.1 Patient Satisfaction 2013 Survey Data From Network Centers

Items	n	Average of Mean Ratings Across Network Centers
Items below were rated on a scale of 1 = Poor to 5 = Excellent		
How long you waited to get an appointment	466	3.9
Convenience of the office's location	473	4.1
Getting through to the office by telephone	469	3.8
Length of time waiting at the office	470	3.6
Time spent with patient	462	4.1
Explanation of what was done for patient	462	4.2
Staff technical skills (thoroughness, carefulness, competence)	470	4.23
Staff personal manner (courtesy, respect, sensitivity, friendliness)	473	4.73
Patient's information was kept private by staff	471	4.3
The visit overall	470	4.2
In general, how would you rate the patient's overall health?	462	3.9
Items below were rated on a scale of 1 = Definitely not to 4 = Definitely yes		
Did your health care provider give you or the patient seen today information to improve your (his/her) health?	457	3.5
How confident do you feel about managing your (his/her) health?	466	3.6
Would you recommend this health center to your family or friends?	465	3.7

surveys, providers often miss important information and a narrative that cannot be captured by the survey numbers. Focus groups have been used for at least 30 years in a variety of settings to encourage participant discussion of issues that are not captured on surveys, and they often reveal very important information.

THE FOCUS GROUP

After institutional review board approval to conduct this focus group was obtained, community advisory board members from the five NMHCs that comprised the network were recruited to participate in a focus group discussion about their areas of satisfaction and dissatisfaction with the health center where they received services and about areas for improvement. There were five participants in the group, four women and one man, representing three of the centers. Each participant was a current patient, and the number of years each had been a patient in the center ranged from 2 to 19. The participants had a combined 33 years of experience as NMHC patients.

Satisfaction With Services Received in the Centers

These participants were overwhelmingly positive about the centers where they received care. In fact, all of the focus group participants said that over the time they had been going to their centers, they had referred many other people there. Specific aspects of the care they discussed included (a) the warm, comfortable, welcoming feeling they felt in the centers; (b) the respect staff felt and observed for patients as individuals, regardless of their circumstances in life, particularly their insurance status; (c) the amount of time practitioners spent with them; (d) the comprehensive, individualized care they received; and (e) the willingness of the staff to accommodate their schedules.

The Center Makes You Feel at Home
In talking about her NMHC experiences, one participant described the staff thus: "They try to make you feel like family there, the reception is great." Another added, "They make you feel at home…it's a nice setting…informative…it has pamphlets on different ways to deal with illnesses….They have a TV playing in the lobby…with all kinds of information in it about a broad range of topics." For most individuals in the group, the health centers they used were located within their home communities, often within walking distance, and were a part of the community. One participant described the center as doing "tremendous work in our community," addressing a broad range of health care needs for residents of all ages, "physicals, teenagers, even STDs."

The Center Cares About You and Respects You, Even if You Are Uninsured

The staff attitudes toward the uninsured were very important to this group. One participant's comment captured the group's discussion and sentiments: "The center helps people from all walks of life. There's a lot of different situations…homeless, from prison, no insurance, and just regular, whatever… they take care of everybody."

Several of the participants had been uninsured or without health care coverage at some point during the time they had been going to their centers, and all agreed that in spite of having no insurance, they were welcomed and treated the same as they had been when they had been insured. Several observed that this was often not the case with other health care providers. One participant had recently lost her health insurance when she was between jobs and was reluctant to go to the center, even when she got sick, explaining:

> You know I felt bad about it, not having any health insurance, but when I did decide to go [to the health center], the person there, she tells me "Don't feel bad about that, you're always welcome…we would never turn you away."…And they never turned me away. [Furthermore, when she did go, she felt]…No discrepancy…no look down on as "Oh, she doesn't have insurance or oh, she can sit here and wait longer 'cause she doesn't have insurance and I'll wait on those who do." You get waited on according to your signature, your sign-in, not according to your insurance or your height, weight, or your color. Nothing like that.…It's always professional, it's always warm.…They welcome you when you come into the health clinic.

The Care Provided in the Center Is Comprehensive, Thorough, and Unhurried

All of the participants agreed that the care they received in the centers was thorough and that the practitioners took as much time as needed. One of the participants explained that at the hospital clinics, you can only be seen on certain days, and "they make sure they [the doctors] don't do anything over fifteen minutes.…They average eight and a half." This was in contrast to the experience described by one of the participants when she first visited the NMHC where she had been a patient for many years:

> She [the NP] kept me in there for hours…and I was complaining (not to nobody in the clinic, just myself) wonder what she is doing…I ain't coming back here no more…but she was keeping me in there so long, she knew my whole history…after I got home, I was thinking like it was kind of good she was taking all that time with me.…

Prior to going to the health center, this woman had been seeing a physician in the community who would "always just ask me what I wanted, instead of me sitting and him going through my heart rate and all like that, he just ask me 'what you want this week?'...He never really examined me....He said I had an ulcer, and all the time I was taking these pills for the ulcer...," but the stomach pain never went away. The nurse practitioner she saw sent her to the hospital for diagnostic studies, which revealed gallstones. "It wasn't a week later I was in the hospital and I got that operation and everything was ok. He [the doctor] wasn't listening to me and giving me the right stuff...I needed that operation real bad, but I didn't know that."

Sources of Dissatisfaction

Extended Telephone Hold Times

Although this was not a problem for all of the participants because some had learned how to maneuver around the phone system by calling a specific practitioner or center staff member's direct extension, several had experienced being placed on hold for a very long time when calling the center. The network administration was very aware of this issue, and noted it on the patient satisfaction survey. At the time of the group, plans were underway to address this by implementing a telephone call center that would triage calls, thereby minimizing the hold time. One of the participants suggested that in the meantime, staff could tell patients that they might be on hold for a while and make arrangements to call the patient back.

For the most part, the group could recall only a couple of instances when they heard anyone express dissatisfaction with care received in the center, and they believed that there were probably reasons for that. One woman explained that she had heard of situations where people were dissatisfied with their care because "they come with an attitude, you know they already have an attitude...they're disgruntled all the time and they just don't want to try and make it happen...when they get to see the nurse, they come out nasty and...they just never coming back here again."

Time Waiting to See the Nurse Practitioner

A couple of the group participants explained that they sometimes had to wait a while in the exam room to see the nurse practitioner, but in general this was not something that bothered them; however, on the patient satisfaction survey, this item did consistently receive one of the lower scores. One woman said that she sometimes took a nap while she was waiting, and another explained that she was relieved just to be there because "once you get there, there's people inside can help you, nurses and so forth, if you have a problem."

Suggested Areas for Improvement

In addition to the recommendation for changes to the phone system to minimize callers' phone wait times, the group participants had a few suggestions for improving the overall care: greater sensitivity to protecting patients' privacy, enhanced staff sensitivity to cultural differences, and the availability of a male health care provider.

Protecting Patients' Privacy

Although most of the group had not experienced a situation in which they felt their privacy had been compromised, one woman explained that sometimes when she was in the center, she "used to hear little buzzes about people, information that I wouldn't necessarily want to hear you know....There is information I heard several times that I probably shouldn't have heard...and probably because I've been in the health care field, I know what some people might not think is personal business, some of those things might be personal business....Makes me feel like sometimes that some of my business might be out there." She recommended that staff have training not just once but several times a year on the rules about protecting patients' privacy.

Another aspect of patient privacy that the group discussed was the nonverbal indicators that might suggest a patient had a particular medical problem or need. For example, some of the group had observed that when patients walked out of an exam room with a brown paper bag, it meant they had either gotten condoms or some sort of medication. And depending on the particular room they walked out of, it might mean they were being seen for treatment of a sexually transmitted disease (STD). Conversely, if patients walked out with white plastic bags, those were usually "give-aways" from the nurse (e.g., samples or health education materials). The group was not able to suggest a more neutral carrier for these sorts of items, but they were concerned about others in the waiting areas having an "open imagination" about the contents of the brown paper bags.

Cultural Differences

Although the group was in agreement that patients, regardless of their circumstances or backgrounds, were treated with respect in the centers, one woman had observed that at times staff could be more aware of cultural differences among their patients. Of particular concern to her were tendencies she had sometimes seen of staff to push some patients off to coworkers from backgrounds similar to the patients'. There were certain religious practices of which staff should be aware and sometimes opportunities for staff to explain to people from other cultures about customs in this country, for example, the practice of wearing deodorant.

Availability of a Male Practitioner

At the present time, almost all of the nurse practitioners in the network centers are women. One of the women participants suggested that having a male nurse practitioner available might make men more comfortable and possibly bring more male patients into the centers: "It might make males more comfortable coming in to get their selves checked...certain things, males might feel more comfortable having it checked you know by another male than a woman."

Using Paper-and-Pencil Surveys to Assess Patient Satisfaction

As mentioned previously, the network currently uses a paper-and-pencil survey questionnaire that was originally developed and available through the Medical Outcomes Trust. This is a 1-page, 14-item questionnaire that is completed after the patient has been seen by the practitioner and handed in to the receptionist prior to leaving. What is currently being recommended by many national groups is the much longer Consumer Assessment of Healthcare Providers and Systems (CAHPS) primary care patient satisfaction survey (Browne et al., 2010). The CAHPS survey is a five-page questionnaire that requires completion outside of the clinic. When the survey currently in use and the CAHPS primary care survey were reviewed by the focus group, the group recommended continued use of the shorter survey, which has, in addition to the questions asked, space to add comments.

Given a choice between the two forms, all participants would choose the shorter one for several reasons. It is shorter and takes less time to complete. As several members of the group commented, by the time patients have been seen and are ready to check out, they have usually been in the clinic for quite some time and are often in a hurry to get home or to work or to pick up their children. Being asked to complete a long form, in addition to being an inconvenience, might also result in mistakes, as one participant said, "by you not reading it as thoroughly as you would by one sheet," adding, "If this information, this one page is anywhere near what it is on this five pages, then I'm first paging it." The group heartily agreed. Other issues people might have, such as poor eyesight, memory problems, or difficulty writing or reading, could be impediments to completing any form and result in embarrassment, but they would be magnified when the same people were asked to complete a much longer form. This focus group also indicated that they never complete telephone surveys or ones that are mailed to their homes.

CONCLUSION

Both the results of the annual patient satisfaction surveys conducted by this network and the focus group findings were consistent in suggesting that the NMHC patients are highly satisfied with the care received in the centers. Importantly, they feel respected and comfortable and believe that they receive high-quality care. Although these focus group findings are limited by the small number of participants and by their obvious commitment to the centers, given their membership on the community advisory boards, the high degree of satisfaction expressed nonetheless mirrored the patient satisfaction data obtained from the annual surveys. However, their recommendations for improving services, for example, ongoing staff training about maintaining patient privacy, enhancing cultural sensitivity, and the availability of a male practitioner, had not appeared in the annual surveys. These were important suggestions that might not have ever emerged from a survey alone, underscoring the importance of combining qualitative data obtained from focus groups and/or interviews with quantitative data.

Although the degree of patient satisfaction with a health care provider is not necessarily an indication of the quality of care provided, creating a health center where patients feel respected, cared for, and comfortable is a first step in addressing the health care needs of underserved populations such as those served by these centers.

REFERENCES

Browne, K., Roseman, D., Shaller, D., & Edgman-Levitan, S. (2010). Measuring patient experience as a strategy for improving primary care. *Health Affairs, 29*(5), 921–925. doi:10.1377/hlthaff.2010.0238

Michael, M., Schaffer, S. D., Egan, P. L., Little, B. B., & Pritchard, P. S. (2013). Improving wait times and patient satisfaction in primary care. *Journal for Healthcare Quality, 35*(2), 50–60. doi:10.1111/jhq.12004

Roblin, D. W., Becker, E. R., Adams, E. K., Howard, D. H., & Roberts, M. H. (2004). Patient satisfaction with primary care: Does type of practitioner matter? *Medical Care, 42*(6), 579–590.

CHAPTER 8

Providing Behavioral Health Care Within Nurse-Managed Health Clinics: A Journey Toward Full Integration—The Abbottsford Falls Community Health Center

Donna L. Torrisi

1992: A COMMITMENT TO BEHAVIORAL HEALTH FROM THE START

The Family Practice and Counseling Network's (FPCN's) Abbottsford Falls community health center, a public housing-based federally qualified health center (FQHC), opened for business in July 1992. It was nestled in the center of the Abbottsford public housing development, where it occupied an area formerly known as "piper's row" because of its infestation of drugs and drug dealers. Among the health center's 11 staff was a psychologist, a South African woman, who manifested behaviors that exemplified her belief in the need for strong community connections. She was the first person to be hired, evidence of the director's commitment to behavioral health (BH) care. The director believed that people did not have the resources to tend to their personal medical needs or their families if they were depressed, substance abusers, or afflicted with a mental illness. Furthermore, the rates of trauma, substance abuse, and mental illness were disproportionately high among public housing residents. A strong and supportive relationship was built between the center's psychologist and the community, and a drug and alcohol support group met weekly. By the second year, the center held two licenses, from the state offices of mental health and of drugs and alcohol. Care provided by a part-time psychiatrist augmented the department's service options.

1994–2000: THE GROWTH OF OUTPATIENT BH SERVICES

As FPCN's health centers grew to serve more people, so did the size and complexity of the outpatient BH department, which currently serves over 700 patients. The ever-growing waiting list compelled FPCN to continue to hire more clinical staff. Today, there are 20 licensed therapists at the three Philadelphia sites. Long waiting lists meant long waiting periods for patients as they treaded water or deteriorated before they could receive attention for their BH needs. Long wait lists also frustrated the primary care providers (PCPs), who longed to see their patients served. The frustration grew to a point of tension between PCPs and their mental health clinical counterparts. They questioned the relevance of a BH system that was not available when needed. Constant comparisons to primary care were made by the PCPs, who saw themselves as very accessible and who treated everyone with an urgent need within 48 hours, in contrast to their BH counterparts. "Outpatient behavioral health is a great service," noted one PCP, "for the few people who are lucky enough to gain entry." When the BH director touted the superiority of the service—"none of our patients have committed suicide"—primary care had a response. They painted a picture of those in the community who were suffering from a lack of care and wondered how many patients on the long waiting list had committed suicide or violent acts or had deteriorated while waiting for service. As BH grew, the two departments, treating physical health and mental health, grew more distant from each other; they were two services under one roof, colocated but with little or no integration. The regulations from both the local Medicaid payer and the state department responsible for mental health licensing only furthered the isolation and the tendency to treat smaller numbers of people but take longer periods of time. The policies and procedures were rigid, and they took up large amounts of staff time with paperwork and rules about opening and closing cases. Opening a case involved completing up to 30 forms, making it impractical to treat more patients in shorter periods of time.

2000–2009: THE DEPRESSION COLLABORATIVE

In 2000, the health center's funder, the Health Resources Service Administration, offered FPCN the opportunity to join the Depression Collaborative.

The purpose of the collaborative was to improve assessment, diagnosis, treatment, and outcomes for patients with major depressive disorder (MDD) by changing internal processes. Staff wondered whether this would prove instrumental in moving toward the integration of mind and body. While working with a team of experts to guide and advise on process change, the center's primary care staff worked closely with BH to create a clinical practice guideline to lead the way. Soon there were colorful posters peppering the health center that asked red flag questions: Do you or does someone you know feel down, depressed, or hopeless? Have you, or has someone you know, lost interest in or stopped taking pleasure in things you (he or she) usually enjoy? The Primary Care Evaluation of Mental Disorders (PRIME-MD), a depression assessment tool, was integrated into the electronic health record (EHR).

PCPs screened all new patients for depression and were provided with the psychopharmacology tools to treat MDD. The level of awareness grew to such a degree at the center that staff (many of whom were from the community) began to come forward and ask for help for their own depressive symptoms. This brought mental health into primary care, a big step forward even though the payers continued to separate the mind and the body. A primary care diagnosis of depression or any mental health disorder became a rejected claim by the center's Medicaid payers. The system simply did not, and still does not, support the integration of mind and body when it comes to paying for mental health treatment in primary care. The center got around this by using a code for fatigue or insomnia in lieu of coding for depression. The internal changes instituted during the Depression Collaborative are still in effect today, and they provide a great leap toward integration. But the big problem still lingered and, in fact, worsened. With more patients diagnosed by primary care with MDD, more were referred to BH, and the lengthy waiting list persisted and even grew.

2010: THE BH CONSULTANT MODEL

William was a new patient at the health center. He was 48 years old and living in a halfway house where he was also employed as a handyman. He had spent 26 months in federal prison for a felony; he reported that he had posttraumatic stress disorder (PTSD) from that experience and that he felt hopeless and had suicidal thoughts. He was a smoker and was experiencing chest pain. He had no health insurance. The nurse practitioner (NP; all of the FPCN PCPs were nurse practitioners) did a full assessment and engaged a BH consultant (BHC), a licensed clinical social worker, in caring for William. A more complete BH history revealed that he had a history of bipolar disorder, now compounded by PTSD. After it was determined that William was not a risk to himself or others, he was treated by the NP with mood-stabilizing medication and was given a plan to return to see the therapist in 1 week and the NP in 2 weeks. He was about 40% improved in 2 weeks, and he was able to engage in several weeks of cognitive behavioral therapy with the BHC because his medications were being closely monitored by the NP. Also, because he had seen the outreach and enrollment staff on his first visit, he now had health insurance.

All FPCN health centers now have embedded mental health therapists known as behavioral health consultants in primary care. With this model, the patient is seen almost immediately, without the need to wait on a list, return for another appointment, and endure a lengthy intake process. Care is provided in the exam room and is perceived as a part of the primary care experience, and the shame and stigma of BH care are avoided. The BHC is seen as part of the primary care team, shares the same physical space as the PCP, and records progress notes in the EHR. With integrated documentation, the PCP can reinforce the BHC's care plan. Because the PCP is supported by a BHC, she is more likely to screen for depression, anxiety, substance abuse, and domestic violence. Before, a PCP might have been hesitant to ask probing questions such as, "What stresses you out?" because if the patient responded with examples, the PCP would then be facing a patient in need of a more lengthy intervention, and seeing one patient every 20 minutes in primary care does not allow for this. The BHC, when called in to see a patient, utilizes depression and anxiety screening tools, as well as other instructional aids like "behavioral" prescription pads. She relies heavily on cognitive behavioral theory, which is problem focused; there is no engagement in any form of extended specialty mental health care or psychotherapy. The goal is simply improved life skills and functioning and a decrease in disabling emotions and dysfunction.

Eighteen-year-old Tyrone was the victim of a random shooting at his high school graduation. Although he was not seriously wounded, he experienced persistent chest pain and shortness of breath. Before learning about the health center, he made several trips to the emergency room, where he was treated with an antianxiety medication called alprazolam (brand name Xanax).

Ultimately, he made his way to the center, where an NP promptly called in the BHC. She was able to ascertain that Tyrone was suffering from PTSD. She helped him understand the body–mind connection and the physiology of his symptoms, which were triggered by his difficult emotions. She worked with him and his family throughout the summer. With the tools she offered, he came to be able to control his anxiety without its culminating in frightening physical symptoms. He left for college in the fall with the plan that he could phone her should symptoms recur and that he would follow up during college breaks.

Integrated models of primary care and BH have been shown to produce better outcomes, including lower total health costs and more satisfied patients. Because the BHC helps the PCP stay on schedule, the PCP is freed to see more patients. This model provides for better coordination of care and improved clinical outcomes while increasing patient and staff satisfaction. The PCP is operating as part of a team: There is reduced provider isolation and a decreased sense of helplessness. PC and BH providers learn from one another and form a thorough appreciation of the sublime interdependence of the body and the mind. Fewer patients overall are referred to outpatient BH, leaving available appointments for those who truly need traditional long-term therapy.

A 68-year-old female diabetic patient had stopped taking her medications because she was overwhelmed and depressed from caring for her spouse, who had Alzheimer's disease. She was grieving his loss, and meanwhile her diabetes was badly out of control. The BHC was called in to assist. The patient was provided with support and referred to an Alzheimer's disease caretaker support group. Because her depression score indicated that she was suffering from MDD, her NP started her on an antidepressant medication. She was followed closely by the BHC and had medication check-ins with the NP. Within 4 weeks, her diabetes was under control; she was also less depressed and was engaged with the support group.

SUSTAINABILITY

This service can pay for itself if it is adequately reimbursed by a third-party payer. In Philadelphia, the Medicaid BH payer reimburses $75 a visit. This amount is higher for FQHCs with cost-based reimbursement, in which case the reimbursement may be approximately $130 per visit. However, 30% to 40% of visits are likely to be for uninsured patients, and an FQHC is required to see all patients regardless of the ability to pay. For an uninsured patient, FPCN does not charge for a BHC visit because it is integrated into the primary care experience, and uninsured patients tend to be overrepresented in the BHC's service rolls. Even with 30% to 40% uninsured visits, a fully productive BHC should be able to cover his or her costs with income. A full-time BHC salary with benefits is approximately $72,000 annually. A provider would need 960 reimbursable visits per year, about 22 per week, to pay for his or her compensation. A fully mature BHC is expected to see about 32 visits per week.

CONCLUSION

As noted earlier, the BHC model has clear advantages for patients and providers and should be endorsed as a viable model now and for the future. It is not feasible for everyone who needs BH services to have access to long-term traditional therapy when a third-party insurer is covering the cost. There are neither the financial resources nor sufficient mental health providers under the Medicaid third-party payer system. This may be different in a fee-for-service model, under which the patient has the resources to pay the full fee for a private therapist. In any event, the BHC model does not meet all needs for all people and does not eliminate the need for traditional outpatient services, and it would be incorrect to assume that it does. For example, low-income and underserved communities have disproportionate numbers of people who have experienced significant trauma, as noted in the Adverse Childhood Experiences Study (Institute for Safe Families, Public Health Management Corporation, 2013). For many of these patients, significant investments by the patient and the provider are necessary for healing from trauma.

Additionally, for families with significant dysfunction, the benefits of family therapy cannot be overestimated. At FPCN, both BHC and outpatient services exist under the same roof. This has provided for appropriate triage by BHCs to the services that are right for the patient and family. It is incumbent upon BHC providers to accurately assess each patient and family and to determine, in consultation with the PCP, the appropriate service for the patient—in this way, the maximum opportunity for patient healing and improved function can be fulfilled.

REFERENCE

Institute for Safe Families, Public Health Management Corporation. (2013). *Findings from the Philadelphia Urban ACE Survey*. Retrieved from http://www.institute-forsafefamilies.org/sites/default/files/isfFiles/Philadelphia%20Urban%20 ACE%20Report%202013.pdf

Best Practice Models and Nurse-Managed Primary Care

Geraldine Bednash

NURSE-MANAGED CENTERS—AN AVENUE FOR CHANGE AND HEALTH

Despite the understanding that the United States is one of the most technologically sophisticated and richly resourced nations in the world, we also have the sad reality that health care here, despite its high costs, achieves some of the worst outcomes in the world. Infant mortality, chronic illnesses, and obesity are only a few of the indicators of the failure in our nation's approach to health care delivery, which is designed to treat a breakdown in health status rather than to focus on health promotion or clinical prevention. Achieving better health in this nation will only be possible through care delivery that is designed to meet the needs of communities and that is population based and delivered in partnership with the patients for whom we are privileged to care. Nurse-managed health centers (NMHCs) are uniquely designed and positioned to provide patient-centered care focused on creating a healthy population that can control its own care decisions. NMHCs have a mission, which reflects the nursing perspective that all individuals deserve the highest quality care, no matter their ability to pay or their community of origin. In these NMHCs, advanced practice registered nurses bring the full spectrum of providers together to ensure that a team of professionals that can meet diverse health care needs is collaborating and sharing to achieve the best outcomes possible.

NMHCs provide true community-based care that recognizes the need to partner with the communities in which they exist. True community-based care is only possible when the community partners shape the goals and activities of the health center rather than being passive recipients of care goals designed by providers. NMHCs understand that patient-centered care requires putting the patients—whether they are individuals, families, or communities—at the center of decision making in their work. This historical commitment to the communities in which NMHCs exist has allowed care to be delivered in ways that connect with the real-life experiences of the patients we are trying to serve. Moreover, the culture of inclusive, community-designed care includes a strong focus on the family—traditional or nontraditional—as the unique center of achieving health. NMHCs connect these principles of inclusivity, community centeredness, and family in ways that achieve better health.

NMHCs are thus uniquely designed and operate in ways that address this nation's most significant health problems, working with the most underserved or underresourced patients while achieving the best outcomes for them. Clearly, these centers serve as a lifeline to primary health care services, but they are also centers for access to social services, education, dental care, and other resources necessary for a healthy life. Their growth and sustainability are vital to ensuring the population's health, and they can serve as models for changing the nation's health care delivery system, redesigning it to ensure the best care for all. The examples that follow in Section II demonstrate nurse-managed health care in practice.

CHAPTER 9

Joining Hands With a Vulnerable Community: The Family Practice and Counseling Network

Donna L. Torrisi and Jessie Torrisi

Nurse-managed clinics are all about engaging the community. This chapter is the personal narrative of the experiences, friendships, and partnerships of one nurse practitioner (NP) who founded a highly successful nurse-managed health center (NMHC).

THE GODMOTHER (JUNE 1991)

"It is my experience that it is the nurses who always do the caring." These were the words of Dorothy Harrell, a resident of the Abbottsford Homes, where we founded our first community health center in 1992. Abbottsford, which was usually referred to as "the projects," was the only tenant-managed public housing development in all of Pennsylvania at the time. Ms. Dot was the president of its tenant management corporation.

Ms. Dot hated it when people referred to her community as the projects. To much of Philadelphia—the politicians and socialites—Abbottsford was where the poor, the undesirables, the drug addicts, and throwaway people lived. It was, and still is, a community in need of caring. This is where we would open our first health center. With Ms. Dot's words to spur us on, we would pioneer a new model of care, one that put nurses at the heart of primary care.

The year 1991, under President George H. W. Bush, was the maiden year for a new stream of federal funding to provide health care to public housing residents. When I (Donna) first suggested a nurse-managed model, I expected that tenants would rebuke the idea as yet another example of them receiving the city's leftovers: nurses instead of doctors? But Ms. Dot was powerful and politically active. She is a voice that others followed, which is why she is known as "the godmother" at the health center today, 22 years later.

For the 10 years prior to this, I had worked as an NP at a large health maintenance organization (HMO), seeing patients and providing some administrative oversight for the practice. I loved my patients and colleagues, but something was missing. As an NP, I was often left feeling like a step down from a physician rather than as a member of a respected profession. When the practice was sold, for example, physicians, some of whom had only practiced for 3 years, received serious compensation, while even those NPs who had worked there for 15 years and played a large role in building the practice received next to nothing.

The medical profession is known for being hierarchical, just as those with the most money tend to receive the best health care services. This was my chance to change that: for my future patients and for my fellow nurses.

That September, Resources for Human Development (RHD, the umbrella corporation for the Family Practice & Counseling Network) was awarded one of seven grants to open a health center. This was my dream, my opportunity to build a practice of my own. I knew that I had to apply for the position of director. I also knew that if I got it, I would be in for the challenge of my life.

To this day, I owe Ms. Dot eternal gratitude for helping galvanize the community around our health center, for believing that nurses could do as good a job as doctors—perhaps even better—in delivering primary care.

RECLAIMING PIPER'S ROW (JULY 1992)

On my first day of work, I met with Robert Fishman, the executive director of RHD. "On paper I am your boss," he said, "but think of me as your servant."

I never forgot those words. They became an important reminder of the type of leader I wanted to be for my patients and staff. I was given a desk—no office, just a desk—in a windowless basement in the corporate headquarters. It was not glamorous, but it had its advantages. In this egalitarian environment, I was given tremendous freedom to create a health center where the community got to help call the shots.

In a series of meetings, the community tenant council decided that the new health center should be located in "piper's row," so named after the crack smokers to whom, until recently, the block belonged. In night after night of candlelight vigils, the community had driven out the drug dealers. Now, piper's row was a safe place where residents could go to receive health care.

We renovated three apartments, hired 11 staff, and were soon in business. Our first year, we served 700 people with a budget of $600,000. Soon after, we began reaching out to a second public housing community for basic health needs. We had no exam room there, so we set up a screen in the tenant council office. We also sent a nursing student door to door with two coolers: one full of immunizations, the other full of popsicles.

In those days, the buildings were in bad shape; it was not out of the ordinary to see a hose dangling from a window because the plumbing inside had gone bad. We quickly became advocates of the city for those who lived there. What good is immunizing your baby or getting a wellness checkup if you are forced to go home to unsanitary conditions without heat, clean water, or access to healthy food?

Ms. Walston is one patient I will never forget. She was 72, and she had not been out of bed in 4 years. Her bedding was covered with newspapers, and twice a day an aide came to change the paper. She was obese, and she suffered from severe arthritis of the knees. We brought in a physical therapist to see her and, with her consent, had her admitted to a rehabilitation facility.

With aggressive treatment, she learned to walk again—she was no longer confined to her bed. Patients like her kept me up at night; could we ever make enough of a difference in a place that had been neglected for so long? They inspired me to keep going.

When Ms. Walston came, literally standing on her own two feet, to the party celebrating the first anniversary of our health center, my jaw nearly dropped.

THE UNSTEADY STEPS OF EXPANSION (1994 AND 1995)

On paper, our nurse-managed experiment was very successful. During a meeting with the medical director of the local emergency room (ER), he told me how great it was: Patients were no longer coming to the ER for primary care.

The proof was in the latest census numbers. For years, the people of Abbottsford would go to the ER for any health care need. Whether it was a bad cold, a persistent ache or pain, a chronic condition like diabetes, or a genuine emergency like a heart attack or wound, they simply had nowhere else to go, and now they did. That was the good news.

The bad news, ironically, was that with the census numbers down, the director of the ER feared that we risked losing funding. While many people were and remain devoted to bringing primary care to housing projects, for some bureaucrats, the real motivation to support our project was so that poor people would stop clogging ERs and taking precious resources away from other communities.

Fortunately, this did not come to pass. Instead, the Independence Foundation—a much-valued partner to this day—gave us funding to renovate an old locksmith shop and open our second community health center in Schuylkill Falls, Philadelphia, in 1994.

Winning over the community, however, was not so simple. Many do-gooders had come and gone before us. The community often felt they were guinea pigs in someone's experiment. Rumors abounded about us being an HIV clinic or drug addiction facility. This always perplexed me since Schuylkill Falls was small—about 800 households—and we had three full-time resident outreach workers whose job was to inform the community about our services.

Our sole aim was to improve community health, but a long history of mistrust had built up between the public housing residents and the city over the years. This was simply part of the burden we inherited. And if the community did not trust us, how could we get them to come see us, much less follow our suggestions for care?

Take Ms. Connie, for example. She had diabetes and hypertension, and each time she came to see me, her blood sugar and blood pressure were dangerously high. I spoke to her repeatedly about the importance of taking her medication, but she never stayed on her regimen for long. Finally, out of frustration, I wrote her a letter explaining that I felt I was failing her and perhaps someone else might be more successful. She became angry and stopped coming to the practice altogether.

Four months later, she came into the clinic dragging one leg. The left side of her face was drooping and she was unable to speak intelligibly. Later, on a visit to the hospital, she told me how her family did not trust Western medicine. She had grown up in the Deep South; as a little girl, when she was ill, her grandmother picked roots from their yard to heal her. Now, barely able to speak, she said, "I wish I had listened to you."

I, on the other hand, wished I had listened hard enough to ask more questions. In nursing school, we learned the relationship between many plants and modern medicines. I could have explained that to Ms. Connie, or perhaps just hearing her out would have made her trust me more. In retrospect, meeting halfway did not seem like it should have been so hard. But it was too late now.

For every Ms. Walston, there is a Ms. Connie, someone I knew exactly how to help but could not reach. Trust is, and will likely always be, the most powerful ingredient when it comes to giving effective care.

THE POLITICAL PITFALLS OF CHANGE (MARCH 1995)

In the mid-1990s in Pennsylvania, Medicaid became managed care. This meant the state now defined a primary care provider (PCP) as a physician, excluding NPs. This was potentially fatal for our health centers, which depended on nurse-delivered primary care.

We soon received a call from Health Partners, a prominent Medicaid provider and one of our main partners, that our contract was being called into question by the state government. Though there had been bipartisan federal support for our health centers, first under President Bush and then under President Bill Clinton, Pennsylvania's politicians were not always so supportive. Giving NPs privileges and responsibilities that had previously belonged only to doctors—like writing prescriptions—took a certain liberal, or at least pragmatic, leap of faith.

As I hung up the phone, my heart sank. There was simply no way to continue what we had started if NPs no longer "counted" as PCPs. I quickly contacted the director of Pennsylvania's Department of Health and the Regional Nursing Centers Consortium to see what could be done.

A large gathering was being organized for April at the Department of Health. Physicians from around the state had been invited to weigh in on the question of whether NPs should be allowed to practice independently.

We went armed with petitions from our patients, and many of us gave testimony. The discussion was heated, to put it mildly. The state decided to study the issue for the next 30 days and then give its answer on whether NPs would be included as primary caregivers.

On the thirtieth night, I met with my women's meditation group. As I nervously shared what was about to happen, we decided to hold the Department of Health director in our prayer circle. The decision was almost exclusively in his hands...or so it seemed.

He called me the next day, sounding very defeated. He was being transferred to another department. It was a demotion in his mind, but in mine, it was a prayer answered: The person who would be taking his job asked us to help write the exception to Medicaid law so that we would be able to keep our health centers open.

A LESSON IN HUMILITY (JANUARY 1997)

Five years after we opened Abbottsford Health Center, word was starting to get out, and we continued to serve more and more patients. Guests came from as far as Korea and New Zealand to observe our innovative model of care. Best of all, NMHCs started to spring up across Philadelphia. We were part of a movement that was receiving international acclaim. Hiring as many people as we could from within the communities we served was a key part of our mission from the start. After all, it was not just that health care people lacked in public housing projects. It was jobs and economic opportunity. Poverty, I have heard it said, is the most fatal disease of them all.

At Abbottsford, we tried to hire everyone we could—from the receptionist to the drivers and outreach workers—from within. But managing all those staff, many of whom did not have much if any job preparation or formal education, was excruciating at times.

Learning that not everyone would be able to succeed, and that it was worth trying to make it work anyway, has been perhaps my hardest lesson as director of the health centers. I was often fraught with anxiety that I would fail to do right by the community and its leaders. I wanted everything to be perfect. This naïve ideal, that I could avoid making mistakes, came crashing down in 1997 when I fired a resident staff member for taking a patient's disability money. She had been recommended by one of the leaders of the tenant council, who took my actions personally. I similarly took her attacks personally.

Things quickly escalated. There were grievance hearings held against me, and attempts to turn other community leaders against the decision I had made. Once I even walked into an ambush: I thought I was going to a meeting about health center services, only to find a handpicked group of people on the other side of the door waiting to confront me about the firing.

This is how I learned humility, and that whether right or wrong, in these situations, it is always more important to listen than to defend. With time, we have both been able to move past this event. The tenant council leader continues to serve on my board. She has even come to me for her health care for the past 10 years.

I, for my part, became wiser and more sensitized to the often countless, untold hurts and injustices that many of the people I work with have experienced to get to where they are today. I often feel like, as part of my job, I am getting a crash course on what life is like for people living in poverty. It is a problem bigger than I, or all our health center staff, could tackle. The best we can do is to help forge a different future.

SHOOTINGS AND SORROWS (1997 AND 1998)

Six years after we opened our first health center, trust was developing. The community was beginning to believe we were there for the long haul. We had entered their lives and their homes, and we had stood beside them in tough times.

One night, I received a frantic call from a coworker. Our community outreach worker's son had shot himself in the head. He survived, but was paralyzed with permanent brain damage. We were stunned. No one had recognized how severely depressed he was. As we came together to mourn and support one another, we realized this was not the first trauma that our health center had encountered—nor would it be the last.

Our leadership team drew up a plan for how to respond to a crisis: Each of us would notify the others. Only 2 months later, I received a call at 3 a.m. from Ms. Pat, our receptionist. Her son had been shot and was in critical condition. We were devastated. Ms. Pat's son had been a familiar face in the health center, one of our teen outreach workers.

As we had discussed, I phoned the three other leaders. We all showed up at the intensive care unit and stayed with Ms. Pat until her son was taken off life support. Since then, I have attended numerous funerals of our staff, our patients, and their families, and I have often been invited to speak on these tragic and untimely deaths. There is little one can say to undo such suffering.

We have hired a support person from our corporate office to help us get through trauma and heal as a community. Though there are huge rewards to serving low-income communities, there is also a lot of pain. To shield ourselves from suffering is to refrain from being fully present.

JOYS (MAY 1998)

That same year, the Independence Foundation gave us funding to bring together the two communities where our health centers were located— communities with a history of feuding and gang violence—to produce the musical *The Wiz*. A former high school drama teacher would direct the show, but the process was arduous as we tried to get parents on board and make sure their children attended rehearsals.

The payoff, however, was unimaginable: The young people worked together harmoniously toward what would be a fantastic finale, and tears streamed down my face as I watched the children who had committed themselves to doing something creative and positive onstage together. Older gang members and parents who had thought of each other as adversaries for way too long sat side by side, sharing the joy of the performances. Animosity seemed to melt away.

It was an unforgettable high for me and for the communities. I often wonder if this experience set the stage for years later when we combined the two health centers into one new space, and former adversaries shared a common space where the objective was physical and emotional healing.

BRINGING BEHAVIORAL HEALTH INTO THE EXAM ROOM (2009)

Nearly two decades after we began our nurse-managed centers, we realized that providing better mental health services was key to our making a lasting change in the community. Addictions, obesity, shootings, depression, learning disabilities, prison violence—these are facts of life for many of our patients. If a patient does not personally suffer from one of the above, it is likely that one of his or her parents, siblings, or children does. The stats are overwhelming, and they are borne out in our health centers every day.

Our traditional outpatient behavioral health service always had a long waiting list. Those who got into therapy—roughly 700 patients a year, a small percentage of those who sought care—tended to stay in therapy, but the rest were left to fend for themselves. As one of my colleagues noted, "The service is great for the few people who can gain entry to it."

For us, the solution has been to integrate mental health therapists into primary care. The therapists, or behavioral health consultants (BHCs), come into the exam room while the patient is being seen. This normalizes the process of receiving mental health care for our patients, many of whom have negative associations with outpatient behavioral health. It also encourages nurses to ask probing questions designed to unveil anxiety, depression, substance abuse, or other emotional issues that stand in the way of a person's ability to become healthier.

Here is one example of how it works. Ms. B. came to see me on New Year's Eve for a postabortion check-up. Her 13-year-old son was with her because he needed a wellness exam and vaccinations before he could return to school in the new year. When I was alone with Ms. B, she told me she had recently been incarcerated and that she had four children who had stayed with her sister for almost a year. Ms. B. now seemed smaller, more frightened, and alone than she had a moment ago.

With her permission, I invited a BHC into the room. Both Ms. B. and her son were able to discuss the trauma they had felt being apart. Ms. B. was able to take in her son's feelings, showing the compassion and extra attention that might be needed to help him recover and move forward.

These are exactly the kinds of experiences that, when neglected, can lead to substance abuse, chronic illness, and even premature death. Integrating behavioral health into our practice helps prevent this. All of our staff receive training on trauma and the brain to learn how to care for a patient who has been a victim of trauma. In the process, we are also teaching our staff about how vital it is for them to take care of themselves.

"Be kind to everyone, as they may be fighting a hard battle."
—Unknown

OUR FIRST RURAL HEALTH CENTER (2012)

In 2010, I heard from Dr. Deborah McMillan, a family practice physician, and her husband, the Reverend Laiton McMillan, both activists in East York, Pennsylvania; they were eager to have a health center in their community. Over the next year, we met multiple times with the people of York, the Department of Health, the mayor, hospital administrators, and the CEO of a federally qualified health center (FQHC) that had been in the area for quite some time.

It was clear that the residents of East York wanted us; in many ways, they were just as impoverished and in need of quality health care as the inner city neighborhoods we were used to serving, but the local health establishment felt differently. I was very ambivalent; the data showed a need for a second community health center, but I was not sure that we, coming in from outside the community, were the right people to pull it off.

I asked for a meeting with all of the players involved in the decision. We met in a large boardroom at the other health center. I began by asking the health center's leaders if they would open a second center on the other side of town. They were clear that they believed there was no need. They were repeatedly countered by residents who insisted they needed care, and the research showed that there were not enough resources in the community at the time.

Three hours into the meeting, we were exhausted and at a seeming stalemate. That is when a petite South African physician rose to speak. In a slow, dignified accent, he said, "Once again, I hear White people telling Black people what they need."

The room was silent, and at that moment, my ambivalence dissolved. He had spoken a truth the others were all too familiar with. It was not that there was no need for a new health center. It was that there was no money for one. At the next opportunity, we applied for expanded funding to include East York, fully expecting to be rejected. But in August 2011, I received an exuberant call from our grant proposal writer. In 2012, we celebrated the grand opening of our first rural health center in a renovated convent in York.

This community is extraordinarily fragile. Mental health resources are so slim here that we have responded to the needs of the people by training our NPs in psychopharmacology and having our Philadelphia psychiatric staff travel to provide services in York. Overseeing a center 2 hours away from our main office takes tremendous resources. For this reason, I would be hesitant to pursue this route again without first finding a director for the health center who understood and practiced our culture and values.

TWENTY-TWO YEARS INTO THE JOURNEY (FEBRUARY 2014)

Today, the Family Practice & Counseling Network has six centers, and serves 19,000 patients a year. That is 86,000 primary care, behavioral health, and dental visits. Business is booming, but ironically, times are difficult for us financially because our uninsured rate has increased. More poor people lost Medicaid in Pennsylvania than in any other state in 2013. Under the Affordable Care Act (ACA), states can choose whether or not to expand Medicaid, and Pennsylvania legislators chose not to, leaving more poor people at a loss for how to access health care.

That means we are now serving more uninsured patients; currently, one of every four of our patients is uninsured. In this climate, it is hard not to run a deficit. A healthy balance for us is seeing a patient base of 60% on Medicaid, 22% uninsured, and the rest on Medicare or private insurance. A shift of only 1% or 2% has a huge impact on our financial health.

This is not the first time we have had hurdles to overcome, however. This hardship has only strengthened our resolve, although we have had to make difficult decisions, such as cutting staff and closing some pharmacy dispensaries. We are working fiercely to try to persuade uninsured patients to sign up for a health plan in the marketplace or for Medicaid.

The future for us and for other FQHCs is bright. Though the ACA has created a controversial stir in this country, it has us moving in the right direction. Health care is a right; anything short of that is immoral and unethical. For the first time in my career, I can look uninsured patients in the eye and tell them that there is hope and we can help. The relief this provides for patients and their health care providers is extraordinary.

In Pennsylvania, FQHCs are making great strides. The Department of Health is proposing a program called Healthy Pennsylvania, which mandates that health plans contract with FQHCs and receive cost-based reimbursement for visits, as they do with Medicaid.

This journey has been profound, and I would not trade it for anything. As we have opened new health centers and the staff I manage has expanded, it has been very important for me to continue to see patients. Working side by side with nurses and other staff, I am able to stay connected to our patients' experiences and be reminded of why we do this work.

ACKNOWLEDGMENTS

I am grateful to RHD for empowering me to develop this model and to our major funders and supporters: the Health Resources Service Administration, the Independence Foundation, the National Nursing Centers Consortium, the Health Federation, the Pennsylvania Association for Community Health Centers, and Independence Blue Cross.

CHAPTER 10

11th Street Family Health Services of Drexel University: A University–Community Partnership

Patricia Gerrity

BACKGROUND

In 1996, the nursing leadership of an urban university led the development of an academic–community partnership with the residents of four public housing developments in Philadelphia. Spearheaded by a public health nursing professor, the faculty believed that this partnership could be a powerful force in transforming the community's health. They envisioned a model of care that was "more than just a clinic," one that considered people's lives, aspirations, and unique perceptions of how health could be achieved. They envisioned the difference between existing care and what could be. Inspired by public health nursing pioneers such as Florence Nightingale, Margaret Sanger, and Lillian Wald, the Drexel University College of Nursing and Health Professions (CNHP) public health nursing faculty spearheaded the now 17-year-old partnership described in this chapter. See Exhibit 10.1 for descriptions of the participating partners.

Exhibit 10.1 The Partners

Drexel University's College of Nursing and Health Professions

The Drexel University CNHP offers degrees in 15 clinical disciplines, including nursing, physical therapy, physician assistant, mental health sciences and clinical programs, health sciences, and nutrition. The mission of CNHP is to offer cutting-edge, technology-infused clinical education that is rigorous, relevant, and learner-friendly. It is one of the few colleges in the United States that includes a major health center in its organizational structure. The 11th Street Family Health Services center, with its large patient base, broad outreach, and innovative model of care, is a primary component of the college's mission, and the center now serves 4,700 students and 6,200 patients. CNHP is committed to leading the way in improving health and reducing health disparities through innovative education, interdisciplinary research, and community-based practice initiatives.

The Philadelphia Housing Authority Community Residents
(four Philadelphia housing developments)

The Philadelphia Housing Authority's (PHA's) mission is to provide quality housing for Philadelphia's low- and moderate-income families by maintaining and improving the city's housing and facilities, achieving excellence in property management, providing opportunities for resident economic enhancement and workforce development, and forming strategic partnerships with surrounding communities. PHA is the fourth-largest public housing authority in the United States and the largest landlord in Pennsylvania. This initiative involved four of the housing developments located in lower North Philadelphia. Resident councils at each development are elected by public housing residents to represent the residents at each site. They are active participants in PHA's management and policy making. The purpose of each council is to identify strategies to improve the quality of life for PHA residents. The councils serve as advocates for residents and encourage improvements in maintenance and physical conditions, public safety, and support services. Each council helps to plan, implement, monitor, and evaluate the provision of services, and each works with public and private agencies to obtain additional resources.

Just 'cause you've got the recipe doesn't mean you've got the cake.

—Quote from a community leader at the start of the project

This statement by a public housing community leader is a metaphor for the many failed attempts by universities and other organizations to develop sustainable partnerships with communities with the goal of improving health. The residents of the four Philadelphia public housing developments were primarily underrepresented minorities, with an average annual income of $10,645 and an average rent of $267. They struggled to maintain their lives and families in less-than-ideal settings with few local resources such as supermarkets and other stores and services that are common in many communities. However, they were not without strong leadership and a fierce determination not to be used by a university. The leaders made it very clear that they were tired of giving their time and participating in assessments and surveys only to be left without programs or even any short-term intervention, as had happened too often in the past.

The nursing faculty worked to gain the community's trust and operated under the principle that the residents should not just be consulted but should also be active participants in identifying and planning health and other services. The faculty provided a safe forum for marginalized community voices, people who had previously had few venues in which to speak plainly about their problems. The faculty and the community began a discourse on solving health problems and improving lives that has lasted for 17 years. This was an opportunity for people who were suffering from health disparities to help directly tailor the design of health care to address unique needs. Exhibit 10.2 details the ultimate mission and vision of the resulting partnership.

Exhibit 10.2 The Mission and Vision of the 11th Street Family Health Services

MISSION: To provide quality, comprehensive health services to everyone it serves with special attention to vulnerable people and residents of public housing communities.

To provide an exemplary model of nurse-managed, community-based care for the education of health professions students and for faculty practice.

VISION: To decrease health disparities through the continued development of the Healthy Living Center model by offering integrated clinical services and health promotion programs in partnership with the local community.

THE RECIPE

Ingredient #1: Listen and Learn

Listening was the key ingredient in the recipe for a successful academic–community partnership. In fact, although the nursing faculty possessed clear data identifying the major diagnosable medical problems, they knew that designing programs around these data would not have driven broad community participation in services they did not design. Instead, the faculty listened first; they specifically asked community leaders: "What do you believe are the community's most pressing health problems, and how could a university and a community work together to create change leading to improved health and lives?" The community leadership responded with an array of unexpected health problems including packs of stray dogs biting their children in the interior courtyards, car accidents where a broken STOP sign had not been replaced, the need for a food cupboard when families ran out of food at the end of the month, and the desire to be trained in cardiopulmonary resuscitation (CPR) for when emergencies occurred on the street and ambulances were delayed. Using their connections in city government and with the Philadelphia Housing Authority (PHA), and providing CPR training through CNHP, the nursing faculty promptly addressed these needs and, by doing so, continued to gain trust and deepen their partnership with residents. These short-term accomplishments set the stage for the next ingredient in gaining input, support, and trust from a wider group of stakeholders.

Ingredient #2: Future Search

The Future Search conference included university faculty and staff, as well as community residents, and served as the yeast in the recipe for partnership success: It raised issues and hopes. This 3-day planning meeting was task focused and led by an outside facilitator. It brought many types of people together into the same conversation to help transform capability into action. Over 100 stakeholders met for 16 hours spread across 3 days; these were people with resources, expertise, and formal and informal authority; the majority of the participants were community residents. This process produced a rich mixture of information and ideas that were acted on because participants felt commitment to the outcomes. Through a variety of interactive processes, they reviewed the past, explored the present, and created an ideal future. The result was a common vision and strategy—to have a health center in the neighborhood that was responsive to the community's needs, where staff protected residents' privacy and treated them with respect. Community residents wanted access not only to clinical services for illness but also to programs that would improve their overall health.

After the Future Search conference, the 11th Street Partnership for Community Based Care (PCBC) was established. The PCBC is a collaborative effort between the health center and the residents of the surrounding neighborhood in cooperation with local schools, faith-based groups, and social service agencies. PCBC participants worked together to identify a shared vision and action plans. Most importantly, they developed trust in the decision-making process. The PCBC provided the infrastructure and support needed to deliver a comprehensive set of services based on self-defined community need. One vital component is the community advisory board, which has met quarterly for the past 17 years to advise the center staff on programs and to share community perceptions and feedback on existing and future services.

At the time the partnership began, there was a record of other organizations' failed attempts to work with communities. In one instance, the community felt so strongly about not having their voices heard that a group of community leaders actually padlocked the offices of a social service agency that was trying to set up programs on-site. PCBC partners believe that the health partnership was successful because it took the time to get to know the community, gain their trust, and form a strong partnership with common goals.

Lessons learned in developing the partnership:

- Form a strong collaboration with the community and show a united front
- Develop and use networks, government, and other personal connections
- Generate short-term wins
- Be flexible and stay cool
- Keep lines of communication open
- Keep focused on the vision
- Be persistent
- Do not be afraid to take risks

These lessons continue to serve the staff in forging new partnerships, expanding support for healthy lifestyles throughout the community, and continuing to be responsive to the patients and aware of the social determinants of health.

Ingredient #3: Space and Fiscal Sustainability

In the partnership's early stages, the faculty did not have a dedicated place in the community, so they worked in spaces identified by the residents. These included an empty row house, a small community center, and two local churches. After the community expressed the need for a health center, and under the leadership of nursing faculty, the university was awarded grant funds for both primary care services and the construction of a new health center building. At the same time, the housing authority received Hope VI funding to tear down the high-rises and rebuild much of the community, which enabled us to build a new health center in the middle of the newly built and renovated public housing. The community advisory board gave direct input in grant preparation for the start-up funds needed to begin providing primary care services through the Basic Nurse Education and Practice Program, the Health Resources and Services Administration (HRSA), and the HRSA Bureau of Health Professions Division of Nursing (DoN). The purpose of the grant was to strengthen programs that provide basic nurse education through expanding nursing practice arrangements to improve access to primary health care in medically underserved communities. In addition, the Pennsylvania Department of Health awarded the emerging health center a Community Primary Care Challenge Grant to address locally identified health improvement priorities and, in the PCBC's case, to expand primary care access in an underserved North Philadelphia community.

The university committed to providing health services at the center for 25 years in exchange for construction funding. The center operated in temporary public housing space, commandeered by the community, for 4 years until construction of the new center was completed in 2002. The nursing faculty provided primary care services to the largely uninsured population. Contracts were negotiated with local insurers that provided some reimbursement for patients on Medicaid. However, 60% of those seen at the health center in the early years were uninsured.

The move into the new 17,000-square foot, state-of-the-art center highlighted the dilemma of how to continue providing primary care services with low reimbursement rates and a high number of uninsured clients. HRSA had invested over $4 million in this program and wanted to see it succeed. With their desire to ensure the sustainability of core clinical services and the provision of technical assistance, a partnership was formed with an existing, local federally qualified health center (FQHC), the Family Practice & Counseling Network (FPCN), a unit of Resources for Human Development (RHD), a large nonprofit organization in Philadelphia. Through this collaboration, RHD applied to the Bureau of Primary Care to have the 11th Street site become a new access point within their network of FQHCs for the purpose of providing primary care and other reimbursable clinical services.

Many nurse-managed health centers (NMHCs), especially those affiliated with academic institutions, struggled to sustain high-quality service provision to underserved and underinsured groups. Although many of these centers received start-up funds from the DoN, they were not eligible to apply for FQHC funding from the Bureau of Primary Care because of academic institutions' board structures. FQHC status requires that a separate nonprofit entity be set up to run the center. Therefore, during the past two decades, many NMHCs closed due to lack of sustainable funding.

In its continuing partnership with the FPCN, 11th Street Family Health Services of Drexel University currently operates a comprehensive NMHC. The FQHC status gained by the 11th Street Center from this partnership provides cost-based reimbursement for patients who receive Medicaid, the center's main source of funds for core clinical services.

Ingredient #4: Health Promotion Programs

The 11th Street Center supplements existing clinical care with integrated health promotion services, fostering a "no wrong door" approach to care. This approach ensures that an individual can be treated or referred for treatment whether she seeks help for a mental health problem, a general medical condition, a dental problem, or another health issue, reducing the likelihood that anyone will fall through the cracks of an uncoordinated system of care. Health promotion programs support the desires of individuals and families to improve their health through embracing lifestyle changes. These services focus on nutrition, exercise, stress reduction, and mindfulness.

The center includes a teaching kitchen where adults and teens learn about nutrition and food preparation. Regular outings to local farmers markets and grocery stores introduce patients to healthy foods and help them learn how to shop wisely. Patients and community members also grow their own food on the center's urban farm. Exercise and fitness are encouraged and facilitated through the use of the on-site, fully equipped fitness center. Staffed by a fitness trainer/health coach, the center is available at no cost to all patients. CNHP physical therapist faculty and students practice in the same space to facilitate patients' safe transitions to more active lifestyles. In addition, the fitness trainer hosts a weekly walking club in an effort to sustain active lifestyles within the community.

DIFFERENTIATING INGREDIENTS

Ingredient #5: The Integrative Model of Care

Every great recipe has distinctive ingredients, even secret ingredients, that make the cake special. This section outlines the different ingredients that developed over time as the staff and community learned together how to develop the most responsive and effective model of care.

"Integrated care" has many meanings, but it most often refers to integrating behavioral health into primary care. However, at 11th Street, the integrative model of care moves beyond these two areas to include nurse practitioners (NPs), psychologists, social workers, dentists, physical therapists, fitness coaches, nutritionists, health educators, outreach workers, creative arts therapists, nurses, and mind–body therapists or alternative therapists. This integrated approach assists patients in making lifestyle changes and addresses their multiple comorbidities.

The center also combines conventional Western medicine with alternative or complementary treatments, such as Reiki, yoga, and stress reduction techniques, in the effort to treat the whole person. Proponents prefer the term "complementary" to emphasize that such treatments are used to complement mainstream medical interventions, not as replacements or alternatives. A guiding principle within integrative care is to use therapies that have some high-quality evidence to support them. The 11th Street Center was one of 29 centers surveyed for a national study by the Bravewell Collaborative (Horrigan, Lewis, Abrams, & Pechura, 2012). The study, *Integrative Medicine in America*, reported on integrative health care trends at centers across the United States and included the patient populations and medical conditions that were most commonly treated with an integrative health approach.

Challenges to Implementing the Integrated Model of Care

The center's NPs were accustomed to directing the care of patients and referring them to other services when necessary. The addition of integrated behavioral health, however, involved much more than just adding another service—it involved a major change in the way primary care was practiced. The primary care providers (PCPs), the NPs, shifted from being independent clinicians to being functioning team members. Each team member had to understand enough about the others' disciplines and training to communicate effectively and design collaborative interventions to meet each patient's needs.

Early in the integration process, several staff members joined the Collaborative Family Health Care Association to interact and learn from like-minded professionals who were developing care models that integrated the mind and body as well as the individual and family. Over time, more disciplines were added to the care team, once again requiring restructuring patient flow, understanding each discipline's potential contributions to care, and a period of adjustment as roles were developed and refined. This integrated model of care breaks down the barriers between professions and provides a holistic approach to assessing and developing treatment plans that address patients' biological, psychological, and social needs. It promotes some role flexibility among team members and requires continuing cross-disciplinary education. Staff found that this model improved both efficiency and care quality and now say they could never practice in another environment.

Given the array of services available at the center, it was necessary for staff to understand all of the services, know how and when to make a referral, and develop written care plans that could be shared by the patient and providers. An integrated services team was developed to address these issues and promote the further development of the integrated model of care. They developed the following diagram (Figure 10.1) to help visualize and summarize the available services.

Figure 10.1 illustrates the array of primary care services a patient may receive. Services are determined by patients' needs when they arrive. Microsystems, small interdependent teams defined at the level of each patient, are formed to meet particular patient and family needs. The microsystem changes as the patients' and families' needs shift.

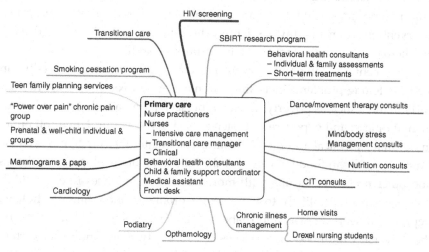

Figure 10.1 The spectrum of services offered at the 11th Street Center.

This model's success is rooted not only in structure and programs but also in *the staff's belief* in integrated care. The provider collaboration through the array of services fosters flexibility, individualization, and cooperation to improve care. Patients are referred for mind–body and other integrative services through primary care to better manage medical and mental health problems and encourage individual accountability for care, self-empowerment, and independence.

Ingredient #6: The Trauma-Informed Model of Care

Why is a trauma-informed, integrative, whole-person model of care important to improving health in this urban community? The patient-centered medical home (PCMH) concept recognizes the need for comprehensive family-centered care. However, most PCMH efforts treat behavioral health as secondary. The 11th Street Center has adopted a family-centered *health* home model that treats mental health as a *primary* component of health "normalizing," including behavioral health services to result in more timely receipt of service.

For patients and professionals alike, the biomedical model alone often fails to capture the vast potentials of healing, ignoring or completely negating the possibility for human growth and development in the face of illness (Schlitz, 2005). As a result, the center relies on an integrative approach to care that puts the patient at the center and addresses the full range of physical, emotional, mental, social, spiritual, and environmental influences that affect a person's health. It uses a personalized strategy that considers the patient's unique conditions, needs, and circumstances and uses the most appropriate interventions from an array of scientific disciplines to heal illness and disease and help people regain and maintain optimum health.

The center's staff grew to appreciate that significant early adversity can lead to lifelong problems including chronic illness. Toxic stress experienced early in life—such as poverty, abuse, or neglect; parental substance abuse or mental illness; and exposure to violence—can have a cumulative toll on an individual's physical and mental health. The greater the number of adverse experiences in childhood, the greater the likelihood of developmental delays and other problems. Adults with more adverse experiences in early childhood are also more likely to have health problems, including alcoholism, depression, heart disease, and diabetes. This fact was well documented by the Adverse Childhood Experiences (ACE) Study, suggesting that certain experiences are major risk factors for the leading causes of illness and death, as well as poor quality of life, in the United States. Progress in preventing and recovering from the nation's worst health and social problems is likely to benefit from a heightened understanding that many of these problems arise as a consequence of adverse childhood experiences.

In a 2008 replication of the ACE Study, Waite, a nurse researcher at the center, and a colleague found that three times as many 11th Street patients had experienced significant childhood trauma/adversity compared with the original ACE Study participants (Waite & Patricia, 2012). While only 12.5% of the original ACE Study participants had had four or more adverse experiences, 49% of 11th Street patients had results this high. Likewise, while 36.1% of the original study participants had had no adverse experiences, only 6.3% of the 11th Street patients had not experienced adverse events. These findings illustrate the potential impact of ongoing domestic and community violence on the children and adults seen at the center.

The trauma-informed model of care that is now formally employed at 11th Street serves as a basis for both patient care and overall organization functioning. It was initially developed for use in mental health settings. However, the center staff has found trauma-informed care to be crucial in the implementation and success of integrated care. The specific model used at the center is known as the Sanctuary Model, a theory-based, trauma-informed, evidence-supported, whole-culture approach that has a clear and structured methodology for creating or changing an organizational culture. A basic belief of the model is that adversity is an inherent part of human life, that many of the behaviors that lead clients to care are directly related to those experiences, and that individuals and groups of people can heal from those experiences. As an organizational culture intervention, it is designed to facilitate the development of structures, processes, and behaviors on the part of staff, clients, and the community as a whole that can counteract the biological, affective, cognitive, social, and existential wounds suffered by the victims of traumatic experience and extended exposure to adversity (Bloom, 2010). The center is currently in the second year of the 3-year process to become Sanctuary certified, the first health center in the country to do so. Throughout the implementation, staff members have engaged in prolonged dialogue that serves to bring to light the major strengths, vulnerabilities, and conflicts within the organization. By looking at shared assumptions and goals and existing practice, staff members from various levels are required to share an analysis of their own structures and functioning, often asking themselves and each other provocative questions and leading to revelations that have never overtly surfaced but that influence organizational functioning.

The staff are now acutely aware of the effects of trauma and the need to incorporate the patient's experience into the plan of care. Creating a trauma-sensitive culture changes the crucial question from "What's wrong with this person?" to "What has happened to this person?" The staff provide a safe place for patients and give them a different experience compared with more traditionally structured clinics. Staff are learning to incorporate trauma assessments into their care and to call on the integrated team to address the root causes of illness and injury.

Some staff were initially reluctant to screen for trauma, but as they progressed in their understanding of trauma theory, they became more comfortable, knowing that they had a team available to address the issues. They began to change their focus from *whether to ask* to *how to ask* about the patient's experience with abuse, given the enormous mental and physical health implications from unrecognized and untreated abuse.

Universal precautions for trauma are now in place at the center. These precautions presume that children, youth, and adults who present for care have a history of traumatic stress that has probably complicated their illnesses, signs, and symptoms. Many providers may assume that abuse experiences are additional problems, but experts who are now focusing on this issue are finding that abuse is actually the central problem rather than adjunctive (Hodas, 2006). The health center is a safe place in the community where residents know that someone will talk *with* them and where their past experiences will be discussed rather than remain hidden because of the staff's lack of knowledge or resources concerning what to do with the information.

> The center takes the nervousness out of asking questions you might not otherwise feel comfortable asking, because it's easy to open up and talk to the nurses and midwives here. It's just a magical place.
>
> —Tanesha Palmer, patient

The staff cannot prevent family trauma and community violence, but they can work from a life course perspective to help build strong, resilient families. The life course approach to conceptualizing health care needs and services evolved from research documenting the important role early life events play in shaping an individual's health trajectory. The interplay of risk and protective factors, such as socioeconomic status, toxic environmental exposures, health behaviors, stress, and nutrition, influence health throughout one's lifetime.

Ingredient #7: The Life Course Perspective

This integrative life course perspective focuses on key periods in individual and family lives, such as care during the prenatal, early childhood, and adolescent stages, and transitions into developing long-term relationships between the care provider and the patient and family. The center has created programs that focus on the prenatal and early childhood periods, with a strong emphasis on addressing infant mental health.

Infant mental health refers to the capacity of children from birth to age 3 to experience, regulate, and express emotion; form close, secure interpersonal relationships; and explore the environment and learn—all in the context of family, community, and cultural expectations for young children. Infant mental health is synonymous with healthy social and emotional development (National Center for Infants, Toddlers, and Families, 2002). A focus on infant mental health is particularly important for children who are born in urban, underserved communities that are nonconducive to child development. These children are more likely to experience trauma at an early age, to have caregivers who are themselves experiencing stress, and to be vulnerable to mental health difficulties early in life. Research also demonstrates that maternal depression impacts children's social and emotional health (Harvard University Center on the Developing Child, 2009).

Researchers now know that the prevention and treatment of mental, emotional, and behavioral disorders are inherently interdisciplinary and require a variety of different strategies (O'Connell, Boat, & Warner, 2009). Of the many possible solutions, expansion of PCPs' understanding of children's mental health capacity has been proposed as one of the most feasible and scalable solutions. The American Academy of Pediatrics National Center for Medical Home Implementation asserts that mental health care *is* mainstream pediatrics. Pediatric PCPs, if trained and supported, are ideally positioned to identify children with mental health problems, triage for emergencies, initiate care, and collaborate with mental health or substance abuse specialists in facilitating a higher level of care when needed. Beginning in infancy, primary care clinicians can nurture resilience, identify adverse childhood experiences and other risks to healthy psychosocial development, screen routinely for emerging symptoms and child- and/or family-functioning problems, and intervene when risks, concerns, or symptoms arise (Horrigan et al., 2012; Waite & Patricia, 2012). Therefore, the center's evidence-based program reflects the best practices and future directions of pediatric care.

This family-focused health care home model with its integrative team approach offers multiple starting points for parents to have their children evaluated or to seek behavioral health services. These points eliminate the usual entry to care: diagnosis after problems occur. Beginning in infancy, the 11th Street integrative primary care team nurtures resilience, identifies adverse childhood experiences and other risks to healthy psychosocial development, screens routinely for emerging symptoms and problems in child or family functioning, and intervenes when risks, concerns, or symptoms arise.

The center has developed a pediatric team consisting of an NP, a behavioral health consultant (BHC), and a family and child supports coordinator (FCSC) to help ensure that families get the assessments and screening their children need. This prevention strategy identifies and ameliorates conditions that lead to mental health problems, thereby reducing the likelihood that problems will emerge. These strategies ensure that children and families have access to screening services that identify issues early, before more significant mental health problems develop.

Current child mental health payment practices are generally modeled on individually based treatment models in response to diagnoses that are appropriate for older children. The payment and reimbursement system often does not support preventive or health-promoting interventions, nor does it fit the mental health service needs of infants, toddlers, and their families through dyadic or intergeneration treatment. The pediatric team understands that children's emotional and social development is embedded in family dynamics and that the social environment is affected by parental mental health and stress. For this reason, the center's programs include a broad range of activities directed at improving parents' health and family circumstances, such as perinatal depression, domestic violence, and family drug and alcohol use.

At 11th Street, all children newborn to age 5 are seen with their parents/caregivers either individually or in the Growing Together well-child care program. Services are provided that address both the physiological and psychosocial aspects of health; they help parents understand the relationship between ongoing healthy physical development and positive behavioral health and the long-term significance of behavioral health support for their children's overall health care.

The pediatric BHC is available to the PCP to comanage patients with behavioral health concerns. Treatment is brief, focused, and based on patient and family education and self-management strategies. It offers immediate, seamless intervention and practice access that integrates care and provides support for positive mental health development. The BHC can also serve as a bridge for children who are waiting for more intensive outpatient care and helps ensure that parents will take the next steps.

The FCSC was added to the team 1 year ago. She sees all women with a positive pregnancy test, and if the woman decides to continue the pregnancy, she signs her up for prenatal care. She cofacilitates group prenatal care with the nurse-midwives, enabling her to intervene early in the children's lives and establish long-term relationships with the families.

The FCSC also cofacilitates the Growing Together group with the NP. These visits group the well-child care program with primary care to provide care for both the mother and the baby in sessions of six to eight parent–baby dyads grouped according to the child's age. Parents spend about 2 hours with the team focusing on development, nutrition, and child and family safety. They learn normal growth and development by observing other children of the same age. The NP provides the well-baby exam during the group sessions in addition to providing care for the mother, including weight monitoring, blood pressure checks, and family planning.

Tools such as The Amazing Brain, designed for the Institute for Safe Families, and Multiplying Connections of the Health Federation of Philadelphia have been created to explain the relationship between healthy brain development and creating a positive, violence-free environment for young children. The Amazing Brain offers six easy steps that caregivers can use to promote healthy brain growth, and it emphasizes the detrimental effects of violence on brain development. This educational tool has been effectively used at the 11th Street Center.

Dance movement therapy (DMT) is another example of both a treatment modality and a starting point for assessment. Directed by the creative arts therapist, a graduate of the university's Creative Arts Therapies graduate program, this service identifies children who need additional referrals or who no longer need intensive therapy; the therapist uses these arts groups as a "step-down" where children can generalize the skills they develop in session so their progress is not specific to one-on-one interactions. Because so many families of 11th Street experience trauma, it is important to note that DMT is effective in helping youth deal with highly charged social issues and emotional complexities, assisting in treating and preventing conflict, peer violence, and abuse (American Dance Therapy Association, 2008). DMT provides a safe outlet for expressing valid feelings, especially anger, frustration, and aggression. The child then has a positive way to express feelings rather than impulsively acting out.

The FCSC also assists women, children, and families in accessing needed services within the health system and beyond. Another important aspect of the life course approach is addressed through its longitudinal perspective, beginning with prenatal care. The FCSC develops relationships with the families and continues to follow them throughout the course of the child's life. This continuum of services and supports also promotes optimal health and development from birth throughout the life span and from the birth of one generation to the next.

The FCSC also meets regularly with community organizations such as Early Head Start, Head Start, day care providers, and schools. These interactions expand the broader community's understanding of behavioral health and create relationships to reduce system fragmentation and bridge gaps in care. She also helps to raise awareness of the need for mental health prevention and to coordinate care for families with complex needs.

SAMPLING THE CAKE: DATA, OUTCOMES, AND MODEL EFFECTIVENESS

Big data is like teen sex. Everybody is talking about it, everyone thinks everyone else is doing it, so everyone claims they are doing it.

—Dan Ariely

How Do We Know the Model Is Effective?

Answering this question depends on program expectations and the integrity of the program outcomes data. On the one hand, primary care practices have specific reporting measures for both outcomes and quality improvement. These are well defined and fairly universal, such as the Healthcare Effectiveness Data and Information Set (HEDIS) measures, chronic illness registries, and related outcomes. Additional primary care data can be analyzed through the use of the electronic health record (EHR). Primary care outcomes data typically report on physiological measures or preventive services and tend not to reflect patient self-report measures, such as quality of life, or the outcomes of integrative services, such as the yoga program for chronic pain, mindfulness-based meditation, and the promotion of infant mental health.

The center was one of eight nurse-managed practices to participate in Pennsylvania's Chronic Illness Collaborative, and it continues to participate in this rigorously monitored program. At the end of the first year, all of the evidence-based outcomes matched, and at times surpassed, the comparison practices in the group. At the 1-year celebration of the learning collaborative, 11th Street was cited as one of three practices that used innovation to develop practices that could make a significant change in patient outcomes.

The center received an award for establishing an innovative approach to working with diabetics with uncontrolled hypertension.

The center was also selected for and participated in the Primary Care Team: Learning From Effective Ambulatory Practices (LEAP) project in 2012. This project, an initiative of the Robert Wood Johnson Foundation and the MacColl Center at the Group Health Research Institute, studied 31 practice sites to identify new strategies in workforce development and interprofessional collaboration. The overarching goal of LEAP was to better understand the innovative models that make primary care more efficient, effective, and satisfying to both patients and providers and ultimately lead to improved patient outcomes.

The 11th Street Family Health Services center has worked hard to improve evidence-based outcomes for all the diabetics in the center's patient population and to implement the Chronic Care Model not only for the care of diabetes but for all patients, particularly those with chronic illness. The three major chronic illness targets of the center are diabetes, hypertension, and hyperlipidemia, focusing on the underlying problems of obesity, which is often comorbid, as well as on the need for self-management and improved nutrition and health education. Using a wellness approach, the chronic care team has included self-management support groups, fitness programs, nutrition classes, diabetes mapping, cooking classes, and a variety of health education and health promotion activities designed to improve patient health and well-being.

The outcomes of this initiative are noteworthy. In the first year of the diabetes program, the percentage of patients with glycated hemoglobin (A1c) > 9 was down from 70% to 30%, heading toward the national goal of under 10% within 3 years. The percentage of patients with low-density lipoprotein (LDL) < 100 has grown from under 20% to 50% in 1 year, and the percent of patients with LDL < 130 from 30% to 70%. The percentage of patients with a blood pressure (BP) under 140/90 went from under 30% to 70%. The data reveal a consistency in being at or above goal on indicators that can be clinically controlled such as percentage of patients who use aspirin, who have had a kidney assessment, who have had a foot exam, who are on statins, and who have a self-management plan. Initiating innovative programs such as an on-site ophthalmology clinic to provide dilated eye exams and on-site podiatry has improved care, supplied much-needed clinical services, and made an immense improvement in the evidence-based outcomes of care. Continued tracking of these data inspire both patients and staff to continue to trend toward goals.

The center shares an EHR with its FQHC partner, the Family Practice & Counseling Network. However, the EHR was not designed to capture the broad range of services provided through the center's extensive health promotion, disease prevention, and chronic disease management programs. A comprehensive analysis of requirements and information needs at the center showed that the EHR system lacked the capacity to collect and report data related to various programs and services provided at 11th Street. Moreover, the EHR did not support providers in sharing their personal knowledge about patients and in using the latest and best evidence. As a result, the center teamed with consultants from the Institute for Health Informatics at the College of Computing and Informatics at Drexel University. This successful collaboration resulted in the development of the Patient Wellness Tracker (PWT; An et al., 2009), a comprehensive health information management system that (a) obtains data directly from patients and staff through screening instruments, surveys, and pre- and posttests; (b) links the information gathered with the existing EHR; and (c) provides easily accessible data for program evaluation across all center activities. The PWT has dramatically increased 11th Street's effectiveness by standardizing, unifying, and enriching the data collected at the center to analyze and evaluate its multifaceted services and programs. The current EHR/PWT system allows staff to use predefined user interfaces to collect and view patient information. The PWT has allowed the center to capture data that were not in the EHR and allows for a more robust picture of patient health. Patients directly enter survey responses into the PWT using iPads. The surveys are automatically scored and immediately available to the staff for review with the patient. The data collected differ by program and include measures such as the Edinburg Postpartum Depression Scale, the Parenting Stress Index, the Patient Health Questionnaire-9 for depression, the Generalized Anxiety Disorder (GAD-7) assessment for anxiety, the SF-36 for quality of life, the Patient Activation Measure, and the ACE score.

As a participant in the Thomas Scattergood Behavioral Health Foundation's Initiative on Building Agency Capacity for Program Evaluation, the center has psychologists from The Consultation Center at the Yale University School of Medicine assisting staff to improve their ability to plan programs with strong process and outcome evaluation measures. The initial consultation focused on measuring the outcomes of programs to improve the mental, emotional, and behavioral health of children up to 3 years old. The initiative has spread throughout the center, such that the staff have developed logic models for all proposed programs. A logic model is a systematic and visual way to present and share understandings about the relationships among the resources employed in operating a program, the planned activities, and the expected changes or results. Staff now develop logic models for all proposed programs that serve as a basis for dialogue. An added bonus of using this strategy has been the ability to harness the power of consensus, group examination of values and beliefs about change processes, and expected program results. Everyone involved agrees on the process and expected outcomes and fully understands the need for consistency and reliability in data collection.

A noteworthy example of outcomes is the results of the center's 4-week Mindfulness-Based Stress Reduction Program. Participants' self-reported anxiety as measured by the GAD-7 was cut almost in half from baseline to follow-up ($p = 0.005$). Using the score cutoffs of 5, 10, and 15 points as indicative of mild, moderate, and severe anxiety, respectively, participants went on average from anxiety levels that were on the high side of mild to levels that would not trigger clinical concern. Notable and statistically significant changes were also observed across the component summaries and individual subscales of the SF-36. Participants showed substantial and statistically significant increases on the mental component summary ($+9.1$, $p = 0.001$), physical functioning ($+6.6$, $p = 0.039$), vitality ($+16.1$, $p = 0.001$), social functioning ($+16.9$, $p = 0.003$), role-physical ($+16.8$, $p = 0.016$), and mental health ($+15.6$, $p < 0.001$) subscales. Nonsignificant improvements were observed on the physical component summary, bodily pain, general health, and role-emotional subscales.

Bridging Services to the Wider Community

Wishing to continue its roots as a public health nursing initiative, the center strives to strengthen the interface between public health and primary care. Public health nurses are interested not only in those who come for care but also in extending services and programs to the neighborhood population, since health is not *delivered* but rather *created* by the interaction of people with their environments. For example, a great deal of violence in the community is often spurred by rivalries between residents, most often teens, in the four public housing developments. As a result, teens from the developments do not come to the center to attend programs such as Teen Talk or Teens in the Kitchen. The public health nurse and the health education and outreach associate have established programs specifically for the teens on-site at their own particular housing developments.

The neighborhood contains one public housing development solely for the elderly and two developments for the elderly and disabled. The public health nurses and students bring programs such as nutrition and exercise in chronic disease management directly to these developments.

Although patients participate in a variety of behavioral health programs at the center, there remains a stigma attached to mental health diagnoses. Additionally, uneasiness exists among the community about interacting with such individuals. In response, the center was chosen to participate in the Philadelphia Mural Arts Porch Light program. The Porch Light Initiative builds a team of artists, service providers, program participants, and city-wide stakeholders to collaborate on a transformative public art project. The program strives to catalyze positive changes in the community, shed light on challenges faced by those with behavioral health issues, reduce stigma, and encourage empathy among community members. During the first year, the Porch Light collaboration engaged approximately 30 service recipients in weekly workshops and welcomed any and all community members to participate in community events including health fairs, paint days, and community forums. This resulted in the dedication of a community mural at the local elementary school whose theme illustrates healthy homes and medicinal plants. The second year of this public art program has been expanded to include children.

Farms to Families

In an innovative effort to target very vulnerable families, the center is collaborating with St. Christopher's Hospital for Children to address the availability and affordability of fresh food in North Philadelphia through the Farms to Families program. Each week, Farm to Families supplies families with boxes of wholesome fresh produce or fruit at a cost of only $10 or $15 per box. Boxes are packed with delicious seasonal fruits and vegetables, often valued at double the price. Additional fresh items including local eggs, meat, and seafood are also offered at affordable prices. Orders are taken 1 week in advance and cash, credit, and SNAP (Supplemental Nutrition Assistance Program, formerly known as food stamps) benefits are all accepted for payment. Boxes come with culturally appropriate recipes for the contents in both English and Spanish. In addition, staff purchase swap boxes to give families the opportunity to tailor the contents to their needs. The contents of the boxes are often used in weekly cooking classes and demonstrations, and taste tests are provided to encourage more families to participate.

The Health Center–Community–Education Interface

You go into nursing school thinking you know what nursing is.

Then you go to nursing school and learn what nursing is.

Then you come to a place like this and you learn what nursing could be.

—Samantha Krugle, undergraduate student

Faculty, nursing, and health professions students have the unique opportunity to apply knowledge in a truly interdisciplinary setting. The faculty helps students to understand the patients and the reality of their lives, in contrast to many clinical settings that focus on only the illness or diagnosis. Two nursing faculty members are embedded in the center to facilitate clinical community nursing rotation, and faculty from physical therapy, the Creative Arts Therapies, nutrition sciences, and couples and family therapy also work with students. A professor in the Creative Arts Therapies department is currently conducting a National Institutes of Health (NIH)-funded research program to evaluate the use of music therapy for patients with chronic pain.

Students learn about the center's community and meet with community leaders as well as representatives from neighborhood organizations. They study the social determinants of health and the factors that lead to a high incidence of poorly managed chronic illness. A unique aspect of their rotation is the opportunity to participate in the intensive care management program led by the faculty. Students visit the homes of patients with complex illnesses to assist in assessing the patients' and families' needs and in planning and implementing a comprehensive plan for care. Students appreciate the opportunity to get to know patients and interact with them to make a difference. One student remarked that 11th Street was his first clinical experience where he felt that he could really do something for the patient and use his nursing knowledge. Students see the patient in primary care and also accompany them on visits to specialists; these visits are learning experiences for both the patient and the student. Many patients do not understand why they are going to a specialist; the student teaches the patient, helps him/her understand the reason for the visit, and assists the patient to ask the right questions and understand what the specialist has said. For the student, this experience creates a clearer picture of what patients actually go through in both making and getting to appointments and following up on visits.

In response to community need, a law clinic was established to give residents access to legal information, particularly around preparations for end-of-life matters. Students and faculty from the Drexel University Law School come to the center twice a month to provide advance directives, living wills, and power of attorney documents.

THE RECIPE EVOLVES: THE DEVELOPMENT OF A HEALTH CAMPUS

The center currently sits on a 3.6-acre parcel of land that includes a community center and an abandoned school building, both owned by the PHA. Sharing the vision of improved community health, Drexel University and PHA have recently strengthened their collaboration and entered into a partnership to develop this parcel of land into a health campus. The university and PHA engaged a collaborative of city and regional planners, urban designers, and architects (including landscape architects) to prepare a neighborhood development and community health center master plan that is visionary, practical, and unique to the community's point of view and needs. The investments of both PHA and the university provide a strong platform for a successful neighborhood campus at this critical location in North Philadelphia. The wellness campus provides a unique opportunity to combine existing services into a unified urban neighborhood place that builds on the shared strengths of community institutions and commerce. Promoting systematic and systemic change to improve the overall health of community residents will take time, involve many people, and require incremental steps while maintaining a focus on the ultimate goal of improved health and strong partnerships within and beyond the health sector. This approach is in line with the National Partnership for Action recommendations for promoting health equity and reducing health disparities.

A major focus of the health campus is the expansion of the existing health center. The center has outgrown its current space due to both the proliferation of integrated programs and increased demand for services. In response to the growing need for space, CNHP led a successful fundraising campaign to build an extension that will double the size of the center. This additional space will increase the capacity to see more patients, providing adequate space in primary care for the disciplines to interact and collaborate with an improved workflow. The expansion will also provide the long-awaited opportunity to further develop CNHP's Creative Arts Therapies department by providing individual studio space for music, art, and dance movement therapies. In addition, CNHP's Couple and Family Therapy program will establish a clinical practice with students and faculty. This will foster the center's desire to provide family-centered care and will include medical family therapy embedded within primary care.

Plans are also underway to establish a community café in PHA's community center on the health campus. This café will serve as a site for job training and will provide high-nutrient, low-cost food for the community. CNHP's department of nutrition and Drexel's culinary arts program will both be involved in this initiative.

A national nonprofit organization has proposed renovating the abandoned school building to provide housing for homeless veterans. This housing development will be part of the health campus and will collaborate with the health center as community partners. CNHP has entered into an agreement with the organization to gain access to two of the apartments to be used to house patients and families who require respite from their current living arrangements in order to devote their attention to their own and their families' health needs.

This health campus will also provide green space for outdoor activities and exercise and serve as a backdrop where community residents can have a safe place to practice healthy habits such as exercise, meditation, and urban gardening. Together, the programs of the housing authority and the university's health center will provide the community supports needed to develop and maintain healthy behaviors for strong and resilient families.

CONCLUSION

What began as an attempt to create a small, CNHP-based program to improve the health status of residents in a public housing community has grown into a center that is now a nationally recognized transformative and integrated model of comprehensive care. The staff continues to refine programs and share best practices with others who are engaged in similar community efforts, and nurses will continue to lead the way in this university–community collaboration. Working with multiple disciplines, they will provide services that strive to meet the triple aim of better care, improved outcomes, and lower cost. Most importantly, they will work together to infuse health care with compassion and joy. Nurses have the recipe but the recipe evolves!

REFERENCES

American Dance Therapy Association. (2008). *DMT Fact sheet*, p. 5.

An, Y., Dalrymple, P., Rogers, M., Gerrity, P., Horkoff, J., & Yu, E. (2009, May). *Collaborative social modeling for designing a patient wellness tracking system in a nurse-managed health care center.* Proceedings of the 4th International Conference on Design Science Research in Information Systems and Technology, Malvern, PA. doi:10.1145/1555619.1555622

Bloom, S. L. (2010). Sanctuary: An operating system for living organizations. In N. Tehrani (Ed.), *Managing trauma in the workplace: Supporting workers and organizations* (pp. 235–251). London, UK: Routledge.

Harvard University Center on the Developing Child. (2009). *Maternal depression can undermine the development of young children* (Working paper #8). Cambridge, MA: Harvard University Center on the Developing Child. Retrieved from http://developingchild.harvard.edu/resources/reports_and_working_papers/working_papers/wp8/

Hodas, G. (2006). *Responding to childhood trauma: The promise and practice of trauma informed care.* Harrisburg, PA: Pennsylvania Office of Mental Health and Substance Abuse Services. Retrieved from http://www.nasmhpd.org/docs/publications/docs/2006/Responding%20to%20Childhood%20Trauma%20-%20Hodas.pdf

Horrigan, B., Lewis, S., Abrams, D., & Pechura, C. (2012). *Integrative medicine in America: How integrative medicine is being practiced in clinical centers across the United States.* Minneapolis, MN: The Bravewell Collaborative.

National Center for Infants, Toddlers, and Families. (2002). *Early childhood mental health.* Washington, DC: National Center for Infants, Toddlers, and Families. Retrieved from http://main.zerotothree.org/site/PageServer?pagename=key_mental

O'Connell, M. E., Boat, T., & Warner, K. E. (2009). *Preventing mental, emotional, and behavioral disorders among young people: Progress and possibilities.* Washington, DC: National Academies Press.

Schlitz, M. (2005). The integral impulse: An emerging model for health and healing. In M. Schlitz, T. Amorok, & M. S. Micozzi (Eds.), *Consciousness and healing: Integral approaches to mind-body medicine* (pp. xxxvii–xlv). St. Louis, MO: Elsevier/Churchill Livingston.

Waite, R., & Patricia, A. S. (2012). Childhood trauma and adult self-reported depression. *ABNF Journal, 23*(1), 8–13.

CHAPTER 11

The Senior House Calls Program

M. Christina R. Esperat, Linda McMurry, and Sally Coates

The plight of vulnerable populations such as rural elders has gained attention from national organizations, as evidenced by documentation of their special needs, such as those reported by the American Academy of Nursing expert panels on aging and on rural populations, the National Institute of Nursing Research Priority Panel reports on community-based health care and long-term care of older persons, and the American Nurses Association testimony offered to the Institute of Medicine Committee on Improving the Quality of Long-Term Care (Rosswurm, 2001). Because of the special needs of this population, it is recommended that community-based care be the basis for health care delivery that recognizes place-of-residence variability. In context, the growing proportion of the U.S. population that is elderly portends significant challenges in needs and issues that face society now and in the near future. According to the projections by the U.S. Department of Health and Human Services' Administration on Aging (www.aoa.gov/Aging_Statistics/future_growth/future_growth.aspx#age), the number stands at 35 million persons 65 years and older, but is projected to grow to 54,804,470 in 2020; this will further grow to 112,037,396 by 2050. Those individuals 85 and older currently are projected to grow to 6,597,019 in 2020 and to further grow to 19,041,041 in 2050. That is, a growing proportion of frail elders will soon constitute our overall population of older adults.

Aside from the growing burden of disease and disability that proportionally besets our older target populations, particular challenges face these groups that will surely place a significant burden on the health, social, and economic systems that society must prepare for. For instance, approximately 40% of patients in primary care practice are believed to experience depression, a widely underrecognized and undertreated medical illness. An estimated two million older adults 65 years and over have a depressive illness, while five million more may have "subsyndromal depression" or depressive symptoms that fall short of meeting full diagnostic criteria for a disorder (Wiener & Tilly, 2002). Especially common among older individuals, subsyndromal depression is associated with an increased risk of developing into major depression. These depressive symptoms are *not* a normal part of the experiences of sadness, grief, loss, or passing mood states commonly observed among the aged. They tend to be persistent and to interfere significantly with an individual's ability to function (Wiener & Tilly, 2002).

The aging of the population will have a major impact on the organization and delivery of health care. In contrast to the fast-growing proportion of older adults, the number of people between 16 and 34 years of age is declining. This portends an imbalance that will affect society's ability to carry the burdens of old age, particularly the growing shortage of health care workers such as nurses and paraprofessionals.

HISTORY

The Larry Combest Community Health and Wellness Center (LCCHWC) is a nurse-managed federally qualified health center that provides primary health care to individuals and communities residing in the medically underserved area of the city and county of Lubbock, Texas. Originally created by the Texas Tech University Health Sciences Center School of Nursing (TTUHSC SoN), the LCCHWC evolved into a fully pledged primary health care center that provides a wide range of clinical and programmatic services to not only the original target population of medically underserved neighborhoods but also to individuals and families in the city and beyond. The Senior House Calls program (SHC) was started as a component of the TTUHSC SoN practice program in 2003 through a 2-year grant from a local foundation. Operated as part of the LCCHWC, it primarily serves the needs of vulnerable elders in the area. There were 5,940 people over 60 in the service area, 18.6% of whom lived in poverty, compared with 10.7% in Lubbock; 2,347 comprised households with seniors (65 years or older). Almost 1,800 seniors were living alone. In the 2000 census, 56.6% of the seniors reported having a disability, compared with 46.8% of the seniors in Lubbock. Many of these frail elderly have great difficulty leaving their homes for medical care.

The LCCHWC established the SHC program in 2003 with initial start-up funding from the CH Foundation. The program was developed and implemented by the TTUHSC SoN for the senior citizens of Lubbock and surrounding areas in response to their articulated needs, which included immobility, lack of transportation, and the unavailability of physicians who accepted Medicare as issues that produced health care disparities. It now also focuses on prevention, education, and mental health/social work services due to identified stressors reported by the target population. While two nurse practitioners (NPs) provide most of the direct care, physicians from the TTUHSC departments provide backup services. In addition, a licensed clinical social worker (LCSW) provides clients with mental health support services.

SHC is a nurse-managed clinical service for homebound elders that provides comprehensive primary care through advanced practice nurses who are employees of the SoN. The goal of this program is to provide access to a continuum of community-based services for the elderly population in the city of Lubbock, as an alternative to institutional care. At the start of the project, specific objectives were to (a) build the infrastructure of the SHC program; (b) provide individualized health, social, and other supportive services to elderly clients within their homes and communities; (c) establish a network of community resources to support the full continuum of elderly home-based services; (d) create fiscal arrangements to ensure the sustainability of the project beyond the funding period by optimizing billing for health services; and (e) implement a quality improvement process for the program. These objectives were met during its initial year, and they continue to be met to this day.

The current goals of the SHC program are to

- Increase expertise in patient pain management, wound care, and managing patients with dementia
- Enhance partnerships in the community
- Provide primary care and chronic disease management educational services to underserved senior patients

SERVICES PROVIDED

The following are the identified services that are provided in patient homes: primary care provided to the elderly population at home by family NPs; assistance with social issues; counseling for depression/anxiety; assistance with prescription medications; and referrals through a network of community providers. The program is operated in collaboration with the Department of Family Medicine and Community Health of TTUHSC, with a designated part-time medical director employed by the SoN. These services are provided during the work week from 8 a.m. to 5 p.m.; telephone coverage is available 24/7 through the LCCHWC telephone triage system. Sustainability of the program is obtained through the following activities: (a) ensuring that billing is completed in a timely manner; (b) limiting costs through prudent clinical decision making; (c) aggressive follow-up on claims; (d) correct coding of clinical services provided; (e) population-targeted marketing; and (f) partnerships with other organizations. Since its inauguration, the program has served approximately 1,100 unduplicated clients who call this service their medical home; because of the nature of the population, attrition is mainly through death.

Each patient receives a health and behavior needs assessment by the LCSW through which emotional, social, and financial needs are determined and appropriate referrals made. Some patients are currently served by the LCCHWC's Prescription Assistance Program (PAP), which provides medications free of charge by interfacing with pharmaceutical companies that supply the medications. Savings for patients during the first 3 years of PAP services were approximately $178,000.00, with an average 7.5 medications per patient. Approximately one third of patients receive psychotherapy for depression, anxiety, and grief. Family support is provided to relatives of patients who are diagnosed with dementia and related problems.

Routine adult services, as noted earlier, are provided to seniors; they include immunizations as indicated, age-appropriate labs, functional assessments, counseling and education that include home safety and osteoporosis care, and case management to ensure that patients have the services they need to remain safe and in good health at home. As the population ages, common themes have emerged as appropriate for treatment interventions with the elderly. The elderly can have very fulfilling and satisfying lives; however, too often, older adults face major environmental and personal problems. In addition, many psychiatric problems are related to the losses, transitions, problems, and stressors of old age. Some common themes in SHC are

- Physical illness and disability
- Death and dying
- Diminished ability and dependence
- Social network losses

- Role loss
- Disengagement and reduced pleasure
- Ageism and low self-esteem
- Conflicts with family
- Environmental stressors

Research has shown that certain types of short-term psychotherapy, particularly cognitive behavioral therapy and interpersonal therapy, are effective treatments for late-life depression. In addition, psychotherapy alone has been shown to prolong periods of good health free from depression. Older adults are excellent candidates for cognitive group psychotherapy. Family therapy services are provided in the SHC program; those needing more intensive therapy are referred to appropriate services.

CHALLENGES AND ISSUES

One of the ongoing challenges for this program is maintaining fiscal sustainability to enable continuation of the program at optimal levels. SHC is largely funded through Medicare since almost 99% of its patient volume is covered by Medicare. Thus, the primary and ongoing goal for sustainability is maintaining a viable Medicare volume to support its operations.

Increase Patient Volume

Several marketing initiatives that are ongoing include gaining referrals from family practice, geriatric treatment teams, internal medicine, home health agencies, durable medical equipment agencies, the Department of Aging and Disabilities, Adult Protective Services, the South Plains Association of Governments, churches, and the community at large through advertisements in newspapers, contact with local pharmacies, and other community activities such as health fairs.

Increase Number of Patient Visits per NP per Day

Schedule NP visits with increased emphasis on acuity. The goal is to increase the number of patient visits per day for each NP from the current five to six or seven. The program break-even point has been determined to be five patient visits per day; to provide a sustainability cushion, the goal is at least six to seven visits per day.

Ensure Greater Fiscal Operations Efficiencies

Create fiscal arrangements that will ensure the sustainability of the program:

- Maximize billing
- Ensure that billing is completed in a timely manner
- Limit costs
- Follow up claims aggressively
- Code correctly
- Target marketing to specific populations
- Partner with other organizations

Secure the Technical Means to Increase Electronic Recording Productivity and Efficiency

This is an ongoing challenge that has been compounded by changes in the information system. We are currently working with the support systems available within the TTUHSC for more efficient processes.

Develop Contingency Plans for Unforeseen Circumstances

Seek external grants related to the social and environmental problems experienced by the elderly population to add to the support available for program needs.

CLIENT RESPONSES

A current patient describes his satisfaction with his treatment thus: "I used to be in the emergency room at least once a month 'cause I couldn't get to my doctor's office. My children work, and when I needed help there was no one to available. Since the nurse practitioner is coming to my home, I no longer have to use the emergency system." Another patient describes her satisfaction with SHC: "I understand my condition due to the nurse practitioner taking the time to explain and educate. I am taking better care of myself."

REFERENCES

Rosswurm, M. (2001). Nursing perspectives on the health care of rural elders. *Geriatric Nursing, 22*(5), 231–233. doi:10.1067/mgn.2001.119468

Wiener, J., & Tilley, J. (2002). Population ageing in the United States: Implications for public programmes. *International Journal of Epidemiology, 31*(4), 776–781. doi:10.1093/ije/31.4.776

CHAPTER 12

Convenient Care Clinics: Lessons Learned From Consumer-Driven Health Care

Sandra Festa Ryan and Sarah Rosenberg

OVERVIEW OF THE INDUSTRY

The inception of the convenient care (commonly called retail) clinic (CCC) industry was driven by the consumer need for easily accessible, affordable, high-quality health care. It originated from a desire to create an exceptional health care experience for patients that focused on individual patient needs and put the patient at the center. The current health care system is complex and focuses on the treatment of illness versus the promotion of wellness, and it was built around convenience for the health care provider. The system is complicated and convoluted and not easy for patients to navigate. With the number of primary care clinicians, particularly physicians, growing more limited, issues of access to care will increase, as will patients' accessing the health care ecosystem at the right level of care.

When the Patient Protection and Affordability Care Act (ACA) was signed by President Barack Obama in 2010, 44% of Americans were uninsured or underinsured (Schoen, Doty, Robertson, & Collins, 2011). Additionally, lack of access to primary health care was challenging even for those with health insurance. Lack of access to health care, particularly after hours and on weekends, presents a barrier to effective and timely treatment for many people in the United States (Guttman, Zimmerman, & Nelson, 2003). Only 29% of primary care physicians report having support in place to see patients outside of regular office hours if needed (Schoen et al., 2009). This often leads to overuse of emergency departments and urgent care facilities for nonurgent medical treatment (California HealthCare Foundation, 2007).

Retail-based CCCs were created to provide Americans with access to high-quality, convenient, affordable health care.

WHAT ARE CCCs?

CCCs are health care clinics that are usually located in retail locations, such as pharmacies and drug stores, supermarkets, big-box retailers, and other high-traffic retail settings with pharmacies, and are staffed by nationally certified nurse practitioners (NPs) and physician assistants (PAs; Convenient Care Association [CCA], 2014a).

Initially, the clinics provided a limited scope of services, but as consumers embraced them and the providers providing care in them, they demanded increased services to meet their health care needs and those of their families. Today, clinic providers diagnose, treat, and write prescriptions as needed for both acute and chronic conditions. They treat minor acute illnesses and wounds, provide wellness and preventive services, and provide chronic disease care and management. Services offered in the clinics include treatment for strep throat, bladder infections, pinkeye, and infections of the ears, nose, and throat; vaccinations for influenza, pneumonia, tetanus, pertussis, human papillomavirus (HPV), shingles, and hepatitis, among others; minor care for wounds, abrasions, joint sprains, and skin conditions such as poison ivy, ringworm, and acne; point-of-care routine lab tests, such as strep testing, urinalysis, monospot, and lipid panels; a wide range of wellness services, including sports and camp physicals, smoking cessation programs, and tuberculosis testing; and monitoring, treatment, and management of chronic illnesses such as diabetes, high cholesterol, high blood pressure, and asthma.

Access, Affordability, Quality

The bedrock of CCCs is providing easily accessible, affordable, high-quality health care to consumers who usually would have to wait days or even weeks for basic primary health services.

Access

CCCs provide unprecedented convenient access for consumers. Today, one third of the American population lives within 10 miles of a clinic (Rudavsky, Pollock, & Mehrotra, 2009). Many of these clinics have flexible hours of operation, with most open 7 days a week, up to 12 hours a day during the workweek and up to 8 hours on Saturdays and Sundays; they are also open most holidays. These hours are generally more convenient than those of traditional primary care providers' offices, which reflects the focus of these clinics on meeting the needs of consumers/ patients when and where they want care. Some clinic operators also offer appointment scheduling to enhance patient access and satisfaction. The clinics tend to be busier on the weekends and in the morning, evening, and lunchtime, reflecting that they are meeting an access need that does not exist in the traditional model (Patwardhan, David, Murphy, & Ryan, 2012). Most of the clinics see patients 18 months and older, encompassing pediatric, adult, and geriatric care, with health care visits generally taking 15 to 25 minutes from registration to diagnosis and treatment plan (CCA, 2014a).

Affordability

The transparency of health care services and medical costs sets the clinics apart from traditional medical delivery systems. Consumers like the fact that the clinics visibly post their health care services, treatment costs, accepted insurance plans, and information about their providers on-site and/or on the clinic websites. The basic cash cost for a visit to a CCC averages $75. Up to 40% to 50% of the people using these clinics do not have an existing medical home, making CCCs the lowest cost unsubsidized provider of care (Mehrotra et al., 2009).

Consumers appreciate the affordability in addition to the transparency. The clinics are able to offer consumers low-cost, high-quality health care because the workflow has been streamlined and augmented by innovative technology solutions so that NPs and/or PAs can provide all health services while also handling some administrative functions. Some CCCs are also staffed with medical assistants who aid the provider and help with patient flow when patient volume indicates the need. Electronic health records (EHRs) and other technologies are used to enhance the patient experience and the coordination of care (CCA, 2014b). Patient consent is obtained to facilitate coordination and continuity of care with the patients' medical home and primary care providers. Most clinics have evidence-based written guidelines and established protocols that the providers use to support their clinical decision-making processes and to ensure the highest levels of patient care, satisfaction, and positive health care outcomes.

Quality

The demonstrated ability of the clinics to consistently deliver high-quality care has played a significant role in the success of the convenient care industry. At most CCCs, standardized guidelines support NPs and PAs in clinical decision making. Used as tools and not intended to replace the critical thinking or the clinical judgment of the provider, these guidelines enhance and assist in the decision-making process. The guidelines that CCCs utilize are grounded in evidence-based medicine and based on guidelines published by major medical bodies such as the American Academy of Pediatrics and American Academy of Family Physicians (Jacoby, Crawford, Chaudhari, & Goldfarb, 2010). Most CCCs have incorporated rigorous quality improvement activities and assessments into the evaluation of their providers and practice sites. Both internal and external reviews are being built into these new entities, for example, formal chart reviews by collaborating physicians and peer-to-peer reviews by providers for quality and standard of care, additional coding auditing, and on-site clinic inspections (CCA, 2014b).

Provider credentialing, thorough work history reviews, and in-person interviewing ensure that providers have adequate experience and knowledge to work in this new independent role (CCA, 2014b). The CCCs strive to establish referral bases with physicians and other health care providers in the best interests of their patients and providers and for continuity of health care within their medical communities. The convenient care industry adheres to all state regulations regarding practice issues for advanced practice nurses and PAs and adheres to all state and federal regulations that apply to operating a health care clinic (CCA, 2014b).

THE ROLE OF CONSUMERS IN VALIDATING THE INDUSTRY

Rigorous research into cost, quality, and patient experience has been conducted by analytical powerhouses such as Gallup, Deloitte, and RAND Corporation. Results from this research have provided empirical evidence that CCCs have been creating a better health care experience for patients. Peer-reviewed publications have shown that CCCs offer a quality of care that is as good as or better than that offered in more traditional settings. Multiple published reports looked at retail clinics' performance against the Healthcare Effectiveness Data and Information Set (HEDIS), a tool used by more than 90% of America's health plans to measure performance on important dimensions of care and service, and each study has indicated exceptional adherence to evidence-based guidelines and standards of practice (Jacoby et al., 2010).

Analysis of costs has shown significant savings relative to more traditional care settings. Some peer-reviewed publications have noted the potential for billions of dollars in savings for the health care industry with the greater utilization of CCCs. Even when offering lower costs, CCCs never lost sight of the goal of creating an exceptional patient experience. Gallup research with a retail clinic leader showed that customer engagement in the care setting was in the top 10% of all organizations that Gallup had measured—not just among health care providers, but across all industries, including luxury hotels, premium retailers, and high-end auto dealerships (Frazee, Fleming, & Rafferty, 2010).

CONCLUSION

With over 1,600 clinics in the nation today serving more than 20 million patients, it is correct to say that this disruptive, consumer-driven industry is here to stay. Consumers voted with their feet, and operators listened to their needs and wants and built a model that is continually evolving. New strategies for delivering care will have to continue to be evaluated, and expansion of scope of services to help prevent, treat, and manage chronic diseases, one of the greatest burdens on the health care system today, will need to continue to be addressed. Continued focus on utilizing and optimizing health care technology will ultimately lead to higher-quality care, improved patient outcomes, and enhanced patient safety. Clinics will need to utilize all professionals to the highest levels of their education and training, with a focus on growing health care expertise in the fields of nursing and medicine, to meet the needs of Americans.

REFERENCES

California HealthCare Foundation. (2007). *Health care in the express lane: Retail clinics go mainstream*. Oakland, CA: M. K. Scott. Retrieved from http://www.chcf.org/~/media/MEDIA%20LIBRARY%20Files/PDF/H/PDF%20HealthCareInTheExpressLaneRetailClinics2007.pdf

Convenient Care Association (CCA). (2014a). *About us*. Retrieved from http://ccaclinics.org/index.php?option=com_content&view=article&id=7&Itemid=119

Convenient Care Association (CCA). (2014b). *Quality of care*. Retrieved from http://ccaclinics.org/index.php?option=com_content&view=article&id=6&Itemid=118

Frazee, S. G., Fleming, J. H., & Rafferty, M. O. (2010). Elevating the patient experience. *Retail Clinician*, 2–4.

Guttman, N., Zimmerman, D. R., & Nelson, M. S. (2003). The many faces of access: Reasons for medically nonurgent emergency department visits. *Journal of Health Politics, Policy and Law*, 28(6), 1089–1120.

Jacoby, R., Crawford, A. G., Chaudhari, P., & Goldfarb, N. I. (2010). Quality of care for 2 common pediatric conditions treated by convenient care providers. *American Journal of Medical Quality, 26*(1), 53–58. doi:10.1177/1062860610375106

Mehrotra, A., Liu, H., Adams, J. L., Wang, M. C., Lave, J. R., Thygeson, N. M., . . . McGlynn, E. (2009). Comparing costs and quality of care at retail clinics with that of other medical settings for 3 common illnesses. *Annals of Internal Medicine, 151*(5), 321–328. doi:10.7326/0003-4819-151-5-200909010-00006

Patwardhan, A., Davis, J., Murphy, P., & Ryan, S. F. (2012). After-hours access of convenient care clinics and cost savings associated with avoidance of higher-cost sites of care. *Journal of Primary Care and Community Health, 3*(4), 243–245. doi:10.1177/2150131911436251

Rudavsky, R., Pollock, C. E., & Mehrotra, A. (2009). The geographic distribution, ownership, prices, and scope of practice at retail clinics. *Annals of Internal Medicine, 151*(5), 321–328. doi:10.7326/0003-4819-151-5-200909010-00005

Schoen, C., Doty, M. M., Robertson, R. H., & Collins, S. R. (2011). Affordable Care Act reforms could reduce the number of underinsured U.S. adults by 70 percent. *Health Affairs, 30*(9), 1762–1771. doi:10.1377/hlthaff.2011.0335

Schoen, C., Osborn, R., Doty, M. M., Squires, D., Peugh, D. J., & Applebaum, S. (2009). A survey of primary care physicians in eleven countries, 2009: Perspectives on care, costs, and experiences. *Health Affairs, 28*(6), w1171–w1183. doi:10.1377/hlthaff.28.6.w1171

SECTION III

Nurse-Managed Wellness Centers and Programs

Tine Hansen-Turton

Depending on the capacity, resources, and needs of the community, the delivery of wellness care into the continuum of care can take many forms beyond freestanding nurse-managed wellness centers. The following are examples of models of wellness care that have been integrated into partnerships and traditional primary care models.

CHAPTER 13

Overview of Nurse-Managed Wellness Centers and Wellness Programs Integrated Into Nurse-Managed Primary Care Clinics

Lenore K. Resick, Mary Ellen T. Miller, and Maureen E. Leonardo

Nurse-managed wellness centers (NMWCs) are practice settings that are community based, directed by an advanced practice nurse, and staffed by public health nurses, advanced practice nurses, and other members of an interdisciplinary health care team. The NMWC model centers around the concept of client and family wellness by an advanced practice nurse (Resick, Taylor, & Leonardo, 1999) and is part of the continuum of primary care. Wellness centers are located in medically underserved urban and rural communities. The type of center and the services provided depend on the existing health needs of the community. NMWCs may be freestanding centers or part of another organization such as a university, a workplace, or a program integrated within a traditional primary care model. Since the late 1970s, in conjunction with the development of educational programs for nurse practitioners (NPs), faculties at schools of nursing have established nurse-managed health centers. Linkages have provided clinical sites for educating nurses at all levels and settings as well as for faculty practice opportunities (Hansen-Turton & Miller, 2006). These nurse-managed health centers actively integrate service, education, and research in their model (Kinsey & Miller, 2012). NMWCs are often part of a university's organizational structure, and the range of services depends on the availability of traditional primary care services in the community and the university's resources. In this context, they are frequently termed "a center without walls" because wellness center staff travel to various locations within the community to provide required services. The 19130 Zip Code Project at the Community College of Philadelphia (CCP), described in Chapter 14, is an excellent example of this.

HEALTHY PEOPLE 2020

The wellness center model stresses primary prevention and facilitates self-care of the individual with regard to health care strategies and decision making (King & Resick, 2009). Most often, services provided by wellness centers are based on the goals of Healthy People 2020, with the four main goals being to attain high-quality, longer lives free of preventable disease, disability, injury, and premature death; achieve health equity, eliminate disparities, and improve the health of all groups; create social and physical environments that promote good health for all; and promote quality of life, healthy development, and healthy behaviors across all life stages (U.S. Department of Health & Human Services, 2010). Achieving the Healthy People 2020 goals requires community collaboration as well as long-term commitments and partnerships among diverse groups (Kinsey & Miller, 2012). NMWCs focus on long-term commitments and partnerships to promote client and family wellness across the life span.

ORGANIZATIONAL FRAMEWORKS

NMWCs are often guided by one or more nursing theories or an overarching philosophy that provides the framework for the mission statement and guidance for approaches to care (Taylor, Resick, D'Antonio, & Carroll, 1997). One example is Orem's (1995) self-care theory, used to guide interactions that promote self-care and functioning. According to this nursing theory, self-care involves knowledge, internal and external self-care resources, and self-care actions that will aid the individual in moving toward holistic health. In this process, the nurse acts as a facilitator.

Nursing care involves ongoing interpersonal interactions with clients. The nurse seeks to understand the client's perspective of the world. According to Erickson, Tomlin, and Swain (1983), the nursing paradigm involves modeling and role modeling. Modeling is the process of "seeking to understand the client's unique model of the world" (p. 97). Role modeling is described as "the process by which the nurse understands that unique model within the context of scientific theories and, using that same perspective of the client's unique model, plans interventions that promote health" (p. 97). This theory stresses the role of the nurse in facilitating, nurturing, and providing the client with unconditional acceptance. Goals of nursing interactions include building trust, encouraging positive views held by the client and client control, affirming client strengths, and setting mutual health goals that are based on coming to an understanding of the client's unique view of the world and his or her own situation.

Services Provided by Freestanding NMWCs

Freestanding NMWC services include health promotion and disease prevention activities that focus on primary and secondary prevention strategies as well as wellness programs. Examples of wellness programs include physical activity and fitness, smoking cessation, stress reduction, medication management, parenting education, and programs focused on disease entities such as asthma, diabetes, and heart disease (Miller et al., in progress). Unlike traditional primary care nursing center models, which provide both wellness and primary care across a continuum of health services, NMWCs provide care that is exclusively focused on the wellness end of the continuum of health services (King & Resick, 2009).

However, freestanding wellness centers are often more similar than dissimilar to primary care nurse-managed centers. Similar to traditional primary care nurse-managed centers, these centers often begin because of an invitation from the community to address health and wellness needs that are going unmet by existing health care services. Wellness center services vary and are determined by community needs and resources and by center capacity. Wellness center staff work in partnership with the communities they serve and are rooted in the core of community life (Hansen-Turton & Kinsey, 2001).

Wellness center staff work in conjunction with the clients' traditional primary care providers (PCPs) to appropriately use services and ensure that services are not duplicated. Although some screening services provided by NMWCs are reimbursable, the lack of third-party reimbursement has been a challenge to maintaining sustainability for many centers that are not supported by ongoing grants, foundations, or in-kind contributions from larger agencies such as schools, universities, or workplaces (King & Resick, 2009).

Deciding on a Documentation System

Finding a documentation system that enables health care providers to document their interventions and track client outcomes in a nurse-managed wellness model can be challenging. The traditional medical model of documentation addresses it from the physical and biological problem-solving approach. The medical model approach to treatment begins with a subjective history of the presenting problem, a physical assessment, often laboratory and diagnostic tests to solidify the diagnosis, and treatment of the identified condition. The nursing paradigm comprises the individual, nurse, environment, and health. In this regard, the approach in a nurse-managed wellness model is a holistic view in which the problem or condition for which the client is seeking care is viewed not only in the physical dimension, as noted earlier, but also in the mental, emotional, and spiritual dimensions.

Community-based nurse-managed models have the added dimension of caring for the client in the context of the community. Issues of safety and community and environmental health are often of concern. In addition, documentation may involve multidisciplinary professionals such as social workers, pharmacists, and physical therapists. Documentation also has to enable data retrieval for measuring care outcomes and benchmarking with other nurse-managed centers.

One example of a documentation system that has been used successfully in NMWCs is the Omaha Documentation System (Martin, 2005; Martin & Scheet, 1992). The Omaha Documentation System has been used both nationally and internationally to track client outcomes of wellness and health promotion interventions in nurse-managed centers. Examples include studies that benchmark the outcomes of wellness models and interventions that focus on the care of community-dwelling older adults in the United States (Resick et al., 2011; Thompson & Bucher, 2013) as well as interventions that focus on the health promotion of women in Turkey (Erci, 2012).

Electronic Health Records:
The Challenges of Documenting Wellness Care

A national movement is underway to implement the use of electronic health records (EHRs) to document client encounters and track outcomes of care. This movement has met with many challenges, including lack of standardization (a common language), variations in practice settings, and the inability to analyze large volumes of text (Hazelhurst, McBurnie, Mularski, Puro, & Chauvie, 2012). In a nurse-managed wellness model of care, EHRs may not be affordable or practical in areas with limited or no Internet access.

Student Involvement in Wellness Programs

Students from various health care disciplines, such as nursing, pharmacy, social work, physical therapy, and nutrition, actively participate in NMWC activities. Participation ranges from community service and learning activities to clinical practicum hours. The learning activities provide opportunities for students to partner with key community agencies to help meet the needs of underserved and vulnerable populations.

Benefits for students include academic growth, life skill development, and civic engagement (Astin & Sax, 1998; Strange, 2004). In addition, service learning enhances students' critical thinking skills as they engage in problem solving with community partners (Sedlak, Doheny, Panthofer, & Anaya, 2003). Within the NMWC, broader implications of service learning include interpersonal, social, and moral development as well as increased awareness of community, national, and global health problems (Hayes, Miller, Miller, & Plowfield, 2009).

Schools of nursing and NMWCs are a natural fit for clinical practice hours. If the nursing center is part of a school of nursing, faculty roles include clinical oversight of the graduate and undergraduate students assigned to the center or involved in related community projects (Kinsey & Miller, 2012). NMWC staff often serve as adjunct faculty members in schools of nursing.

Undergraduate and graduate nursing students have the opportunity to be actively engaged in NMWC activities that largely focus on underserved populations. Activities for undergraduate nursing students include participation in primary and secondary prevention strategies at the wellness center or in the community with a "center without walls" framework. Examples of these activities include home-visiting programs, seasonal influenza campaigns, parenting classes at local YMCAs, promotion of physical activity in school settings, heart health classes at senior centers, healthy eating programs, and blood pressure screenings at churches and health fairs (Miller et al., in progress).

Activities for graduate nursing students include preceptorship by an advanced practice nurse, usually an NP. Graduate nursing students have the opportunity for hands-on experience in the roles of caregiver, administrator, and researcher. For example, graduate students work in the caregiver role with clients to develop wellness plans that augment the PCP's medical management plan. In addition to educating about medication, diet, exercise, laboratory values, and safety, the graduate student collaborates with the PCP to implement the medical management plan in the context of the client's day-to-day routine. Students receive firsthand experience in managing wellness in the context of chronic disease conditions. In the nurse administrator role, graduate students have the opportunity to experience strategic planning as well as the day-to-day administration of a nurse-managed business; activities may include implementing standards and regulations and creating a budget. By utilizing research, measuring care delivery outcomes, and generating knowledge, graduate students gain experience in implementing the nurse researcher role. They also gain practical experience in grant writing and in creating survey tools to measure, analyze, and use outcome data and ways to meet the sustainability challenges of a nurse-managed endeavor.

Initiatives such as these benefit students, faculty, and community participants. Students benefit in multiple ways because clinical assignments at NMWCs expose them to real-life situations that individuals, families, and groups experience beyond the boundaries of the acute care setting. The realities of transportation difficulties, neighborhood safety, child care issues, ability to pay for required prescriptions, and living conditions discovered after home visits are only a few of the ways that students gain firsthand knowledge of the multiple challenges facing many individuals and families in the community. Faculty benefit by having the opportunity to serve vulnerable populations while engaging in practice in multiple settings. The community ultimately benefits from receiving access to primary and secondary prevention strategies as well as health promotion and disease prevention initiatives that are otherwise not available or accessible.

The Zip Code Project Data Collection Tool: An Example of Undergraduate Postclinical Documentation

Quantifying undergraduate nursing community experiences in wellness centers is challenging. One method being utilized by four Pennsylvania nursing programs is a data collection tool that was originally developed by CCP to describe clients served and document programs provided through its 19130 Zip Code Project (see Chapter 14). Funding provided by the Independence Foundation has been managed by CCP.

After each project-related clinical experience, students log onto a Survey Monkey website with a specific user name and password. They then enter encounter information regarding their clinical experience. The data entered are either for "individual" or for "group" encounters. An individual encounter is a one-on-one encounter, such as a home care or hospice visit, or one-on-one client teaching. If the student accompanies a home care nurse to six client homes, the student then enters the encounters on six separate "individual" surveys. A group encounter is documented for health fairs, flu vaccine clinics, and mass screening events. In this instance, encounter data are entered into one "group" encounter form.

No identifying client information is entered into the survey. Encounter data are collected for the date and site location, numbers of males and females, ages and ethnicities of the clients, and the primary and secondary prevention strategies that were implemented. Drop-down boxes appear on each survey page for students to select their appropriate interventions. The survey concludes with a box for "other" information where students can provide qualitative comments.

If students are assigned in pairs (or larger groups) to a community site, the student group as a whole enters the data into the website. This way, the data entry is not duplicated by more than one student for the same experience. Initially, faculty guidance is necessary to complete the encounter forms correctly. The tool, however, is user-friendly; once students enter encounter data for one group and one individual encounter, the majority of them are able to continue data entry independently for the remainder of the semester. The student takes a screenshot to confirm that the data were entered for the encounter.

The managing organization, CCP, has the personnel who statistically analyze the data and share the results with the participating centers. An Excel spreadsheet detailing both the individual and group encounter results is sent to the clinical liaison of each participating institution. This is done on an annual basis, but reports can be obtained earlier if needed.

There are several ways that these encounter data are useful for wellness centers. They provide demographic information regarding the populations served and quantify the types of primary and secondary prevention strategies being utilized in outpatient settings. Information regarding number and type of referrals is also assessed. This information is valuable when writing the background or needs assessment section of a grant proposal. The data also justify additional clinical faculty needs in community settings. Students are introduced to the importance of nursing documentation in nontraditional settings. The Zip Code Project's data collection tool is a valuable method for capturing population-based activities in NMWCs.

Faculty Practice in Wellness Programs

As noted earlier in this chapter, many of the NMWCs are housed in or affiliated with academic institutions, so the individuals who are managing or working in these sites are often faculty who teach in the classroom as well as in the clinical area and maintain a faculty practice in these centers. These individuals need to show evidence of scholarly activity for the purpose of promotion and tenure (Resick & Leonardo, 2009). Clinical scholarship involves quality, governance, leadership, and knowledge development (Fiandt et al., 2004). "The wellness center is a bridge between theory and practice, integrating the scholarship of research, teaching, and practice, and operationalizing the mission statement of the institution" (Leonardo, Resick, Torrisi, Hanson-Turton, & Dienhardt, 2009, p. 29).

There are many specific definitions of faculty practice, but most agree that it includes the direct application of nursing expertise to individuals, communities, and students. As such, it encompasses all aspects of nursing service delivery for which evidence is presented of direct impact in solving health care problems or in defining a community's health problems.

NMWCs provide faculty with not only clinical practice opportunities but also the opportunity for research and other scholarship ventures (Thompson & Bucher, 2013).

Since many of these centers are based in academic institutions, student clinical assignments are made according to the academic calendar. As clinicians, faculty can provide continuity of care with student clinical practice participation (Tansey, 1999) as the primary caregivers. Also in this role, they may function as preceptors, mentors, and role models for students who are assigned to the centers for clinical experience (Resick & Leonardo, 2009). According to Boyer, this is referred to as the scholarship of application (Boyer, 1990).

Teaching is central to scholarship because teachers and faculty design, coordinate, and supervise learning experiences for students. They may also be direct care providers who delegate care to students and, as such, also function as role models. NMWCs provide not only well-oriented health care services to vulnerable populations, but also community-based, cross-cultural health care experiences for students (Resick & Leonardo, 2009). Nurses are in key positions to provide health and wellness services in community settings with an emphasis on aggregate and population-based care (Hayward, 2005). Although an advanced practice faculty will ideally provide oversight for the NMWC, a wellness center may include nursing faculty with all levels of expertise, because services focus on self-care and healthy lifestyles, health maintenance issues in the context of chronic conditions, and general health promotion (Tansey, 1999).

These settings also provide faculty with access to clients who can participate in clinical research activities. When faculty work with clients to promote their health and wellness, they may experience more trust and agree to volunteer for research activities because of the commitment faculty have for them. Other faculty may be more interested in seeking external funding to develop protocols or to do program evaluation as a form of scholarship.

Measuring Outcomes and Gathering Data

Wellness center models need to have evaluation plans to assess the effectiveness of their activities. The evaluation process can be organized into categories. One technique in an academic wellness center model is to organize evaluation into three areas: health professions/nursing student outcomes, program outcomes, and client-centered outcomes.

Examples of student outcomes to evaluate could be student learning and satisfaction as well as faculty satisfaction. Another area of outcomes measurement could be stakeholders who provide in-kind support to the nurse-managed initiatives, such as service coordinators, community senior centers, and housing managers. Examples of program outcomes could be numbers of unduplicated clients who attend events or staff satisfaction. Examples of client outcomes could be client satisfaction and improved knowledge, behaviors, and status.

Client outcomes depend on the population focus of the wellness center. For example, if the center's focus is on clients with one or more chronic illness, one outcome could be stabilization and avoiding hospitalization or readmission rather than improving status.

Data gathering can be done by completing paper-and-pencil or electronic surveys and through focus groups, as well as through chart audits and audits of the numbers of individuals who attend specific events. Once analyzed, data can be used to improve student, program, and client outcomes. Challenges to data collection include the availability of valid and reliable tools and time constraints to develop the tools and collect the data. Intercoder reliability of documentation is often difficult to achieve even between two nurses in the same nursing center (Resick, Hayes, Leonardo, & Plowfield, 2009).

SUSTAINABILITY

Sustainability is one of the greatest challenges of NMWCs. The challenge of sustainability is a common dilemma that funders and grantees both face at the end of an initiative's funding period (Cutler, 2002). However, without the ability to maintain fiscal sustainability, NMWCs may fail to reach their full potential for positively influencing the future of health care (McBryde-Foster, 2005).

Financial support for NMWCs mainly comes from grants, contracts, foundations, private giving, and fund-raising, as well as in-kind support from stakeholders. Grants are the primary source of initial and ongoing funding. In some NMWCs, retired and volunteer nurses serve as key members of the wellness team. One example, from Duquesne's Community-Based Health and Wellness Center for Older Adults in Pittsburgh, Pennsylvania, is the Retired Nurses Working in Neighborhoods program, which has been in operation since 2006 (Resick, Leonardo, Kruman, & Carlson, 2009).

This initiative grew out of the ongoing challenge of staffing multiple academic nursing center sites in Pittsburgh neighborhoods. Retired and semiretired nurses were recruited from surrounding neighborhoods to staff the NMWCs throughout the calendar year. Many of these nurses are alumnae of the Duquesne University School of Nursing and other nearby schools of nursing. The volunteer nurses work with students and other staff members 1 to 2 days per month under the supervision of advanced practice nurse faculty volunteers.

WELLNESS CENTERS AND INTEGRATED WELLNESS PROGRAMS IN TRADITIONAL PRIMARY CARE MODELS: FILLING THE HEALTH CARE GAP

Wellness centers complement existing primary care services. Wellness centers' staff members maintain strong relationships with health care providers in nurse-managed primary care centers, community health centers, clinics, private practices, long-term care facilities, and other organizations (Kinsey & Miller, 2014). Wellness centers also play an important role in the national health care crisis facing underserved, vulnerable populations who are uninsured or underinsured. Healthy People 2020 goals and objectives provide a framework for services that are planned, implemented, and evaluated through the wellness center model (Kinsey & Miller, 2014). The Patient Protection and Affordable Care Act (ACA) of 2010 promotes prevention, wellness, and public health, supporting health promotion at the local, state, and federal levels. Title IV of the ACA, "Prevention of Chronic Disease and Improving Public Health," explicitly states, "The Act will promote prevention, wellness, and the public health and provides an unprecedented funding commitment to these areas. It directs the creation of a national prevention and health promotion strategy that incorporates the most effective and achievable methods to improve the health status of Americans and reduce the incidence of preventable illness and disability in the United States" (U.S. Department of Health & Human Services, 2012).

NMWCs are effective and achievable models of health care delivery. As such, they have the potential to play a major role in multiple ways based on ACA Title IV. Opportunities are countless for increased partnerships with universities, communities, and primary care practitioners to augment care received. Services will not be duplicated, but rather enhanced, with additional primary prevention, advocacy, and case management by NMWC staff. The future holds great promise for expanding NMWC services at the local and national levels.

REFERENCES

Astin, L., & Sax, A. (1998). How undergraduates are affected by service participation. *Journal of College Student Development, 39*(3), 251–263.

Boyer, E. L. (1990). *Scholarship reconsidered: Priorities of the professoriate*. Princeton, NJ: The Carnegie Foundation for the Advancement of Teaching.

Erickson, H. C., Tomlin, E. M., & Swain, M. A. P. (1983). *Modeling and role-modeling: A theory and paradigm for nursing*. Englewood Cliffs, NJ: Prentice-Hall.

Erci, B. (2012). The effectiveness of the Omaha System intervention on the women's health Promotion lifestyle profile and quality of life. *Journal of Advanced Nursing, 68*(4), 898–907. doi: 10.1111/j.1365-2648.2011.05794.x

Fiandt, K., Barr, K., Hille, G., Pelish, P., Pozehl, B., Hulme, P.,…Burge, S. (2004). Identifying clinical scholarship faculty guidelines for faculty practice. *Journal of Professional Nursing, 20*(3), 147–155.

Hansen-Turton, T., & Kinsey, K. (2001). The quest for self-sustainability: Nurse-managed health centers meeting the policy challenge. *Policy Politics Nurse Practitioner, 2*(4), 304–309. doi: 10.1177/152715440100200408

Hansen-Turton, T., & Miller, M. E. (2006). Nurses and nurse-managed health centers fill health care gaps. *The Pennsylvania Nurse, 61*(2), 18.

Hayes, E., Miller, J., Miller, M. E., & Plowfield, L. (2009). Community service and learning and student engagement. In T. Hansen-Turton, M. E. T. Miller, & P. A. Greiner (Eds.). *Nurse-managed wellness centers: Developing and maintaining your center* (pp. 87–103). New York, NY: Springer Publishing.

Hayward, K. S. (2005). Facilitating interdisciplinary practice through mobile service provision to the older rural adult. *Geriatric Nursing, 26*(1), 29–33. doi:10.1016/j.gerinurse.2004.11.011

Hazelhurst, B., McBurnie, M. A., Mularski, R. A., Puro, J. E., & Chauvie, S. L. (2012). Automating care quality measurement with health information technology. *The American Journal of Managed Care, 18*(6), 312–319.

King, E., & Resick, L. K. (2009). What is a nurse-managed wellness center? In T. Hansen-Turton, M. E. T. Miller, & P. A. Greiner (Eds.). *Nurse-managed wellness centers: Developing and maintaining your center* (pp. 7–11). New York, NY: Springer.

Kinsey, K., & Miller, M. E. (2012). The nursing center: A model for nursing practice in the community. In M. Stanhope & J. Lancaster (Eds.), *Public health nursing: Population centered health care in the community 8th edition* (pp. 461–482). Maryland Heights, MO: Elsevier.

Kinsey, K., & Miller, M. E. (2014). The nursing center: A model for nursing practice in the community. In M. Stanhope & J. Lancaster (Eds.), *Public health nursing: Population centered health care in the community 9th edition* (in press). Maryland Heights: MO: Elsevier.

Leonardo, M. E., Resick, L. K., Torrisi, D., Hansen-Turton, T., & Dienhardt, A. (2009). Planning a wellness center. In T. Hansen-Turton, M. E. T. Miller, & P. A. Greiner (Eds.). *Nurse-managed wellness centers: Developing and maintaining your center* (pp. 29–38). New York, NY: Springer Publishing.

Martin, K. S. (2005). *The Omaha system: A key to practice, documentation, and information management.* (Reprinted 2nd ed.). Omaha, NE: Health Connections Press.

Martin. K. S., & Sheet, N. J. (1992). *The Omaha system: Application for community health nursing.* Philadelphia, PA: Saunders.

McBryde-Foster, M. (2005). Break-even analysis in a nurse-managed center. *Nursing Economics, 23*(1), 31–34.

Miller, M. E., Leonardo, M., Mengel, A., Miller, J., Resick, L., Rothman, N., & Thompson, C. (in progress). *Nurse-led wellness centers: The world's best kept secret.*

Orem, D. (1995). *Nursing concepts of practice* (5th ed.). St. Louis, MO: Mosby.

Resick, L. K., Hayes, E., Leonardo, M. E., & Plowfield, L. (2009). Documenting outcomes. In T. Hansen-Turton, M. E. T. Miller, & P. A. Greiner (Eds.), *Nurse-managed wellness centers: Developing and maintaining your center* (pp. 113–118). New York NY: Springer Publishing.

Resick, L. K., & Leonardo, M. E. (2009). Application of the Boyer Model of scholarship in nurse-managed wellness centers. In T. Hansen-Turton, M. E. T. Miller, & P. A. Greiner (Eds.), *Nurse-managed wellness centers: Developing and maintaining your center* (pp. 13–18). New York, NY: Springer Publishing.

Resick, L. K., Leonardo, M. E., Kruman, B. J., & Carlson, M. R. (2009). The retired nurses working in neighborhoods (RN+WIN) program: An approach toward sustainability of an academic nurse-managed wellness center. *Home Health Care Management & Practice, 22*(4), 271–277. doi:10.1177/1084822309348775

Resick, L., Leonardo, M. E., McGinnis, K., Stewart, J., Goss, C., & Ellison, T. (2011). A retrospective data analysis of two academic nurse-managed wellness center sites. *Journal of Gerontological Nursing, 37*(6), 43–52. doi: 10.3928/00989134 -20110302-02

Resick, L. K., Taylor, C. A., & Leonardo, M. E. (1999). The nurse-managed wellness clinic model developed by Duquesne University School of Nursing. *Home Health Care Management and Practice, 11*(6), 26–35. doi: 10.1177/108482239901100607

Sedlak, C.A., Doheny, M. O., Panthofer, N., & Anaya, E. (2003). Critical thinking in students' service-learning experiences. *College Teaching, 51,* 99–103. doi:10.1080/87567550309596420

Strange, A. (2004). Long-term academic benefits of service-learning: When and where do they manifest themselves? *College Student Journal, 38*(2), 257–261.

Tansey, E. M. (1999). The nursing wellness center: A win-win situation for faculty. *Association of Black Nursing Faculty Journal, 10*(2), 50–51.

Taylor, C. A., Resick, L. K., D'Antonio, J., & Carroll, T. L. (1997). The advanced practice nurse role in implementing and evaluating two nurse-managed wellness clinics: Lessons learned about structure, process, and outcomes. *Advanced Practice Nursing Quarterly, 3*(2), 36–45.

Thompson, C. W., & Bucher, J. A. (2013). Meeting baccalaureate public/community health nursing education competencies in nurse-managed wellness centers. *Journal of Professional Nursing, 29*(3), 155–162. doi: 10.1016/j.profnurs.2012.04.017

U.S. Department of Health & Human Services. (2010). *Healthy people 2020.* Washington, DC: Author. Retrieved from http://www.healthypeople.gov

U.S. Department of Health & Human Services. (2012). *The affordable care act.* Washington, DC: Author. Retrieved from http://www.hhs.gov/health care/rights/law/

Waite, R., & Patricia, A. S. (2012). Childhood trauma and adult self-reported depression. *ABNF Journal, 23*(1), 8–13.

CHAPTER 14

The 19130 Zip Code Project: A Journey to Our Neighborhood

Andrea Mengel and M. Elaine Tagliareni

The 19130 Zip Code Project at the Community College of Philadelphia (CCP) started as a curriculum innovation: the CCP Department of Nursing's response to the national shift toward community-based health care. The project resulted in the refocusing of the nursing curriculum and the development of partnerships with CCP's neighbors in the 19130 zip code (American Association of Colleges of Nursing, 1999). It also is an excellent example of a nurse-managed wellness center without walls.

Since it began in 1996, the Zip Code Project has put down deep roots in the neighborhood and in the nursing curriculum. It has produced a community-based model for educating local health professionals and a service-learning model for enhancing health service delivery by local agencies. Dissemination of the Zip Code Project curriculum and service-learning model has occurred at the local, regional, and national levels through multiple forums. Yet it remains a small-scale, down-to-earth program that is well within the means of most nursing programs. This chapter provides an overview of the Zip Code Project and how and why it works.

CCP enrolls some 45,000 students annually, more than half of them from minority groups and many of them beginning courses at the pre-college level. The Department of Nursing has a long tradition of preparing graduates, about 100 annually, for entry-level positions in hospitals and nursing homes. But the national shift toward a community-based system of health care indicated that a curriculum change would be required if the nursing graduates were to be prepared for emerging roles in community-based care (American Association of Colleges of Nursing, 1999; Resick & Leonardo, 2009; Thompson & Bucher, 2013).

In 1993, the Independence Foundation of Philadelphia endowed Independence Foundation Chairs in Nursing at four local academic institutions: CCP, LaSalle University, Temple University, and the University of Pennsylvania. Elaine Tagliareni held the position of Independence Foundation Chair in Nursing at CCP from its inception until 2009 when she moved to the National League for Nursing as chief program officer. Andrea Mengel, who was head of the Department of Nursing from 1996 until 2009, stepped into the chair role and currently holds the position.

From 1993 to 1995, Elaine Tagliareni and her colleagues in the Department of Nursing embarked on a journey to develop an innovative, community-based curriculum model. With a planning grant from the Independence Foundation, the nursing faculty envisioned a range of projects, including CCP's own nurse-managed clinic or a citywide clinical experience. Following pilot testing of a project in 1995, the nursing faculty found the citywide project to be too diffuse. The nursing faculty rethought their plans, reviewing their considerable success with the W. K. Kellogg Community Nursing Home Partnership in the early 1990s. That experience had shown the value of building relationships with nursing home staff and residents over an extended period of time to plan comprehensive, personalized care (Kinsey & Miller, 2012). Why not apply those principles to community experiences by returning to the same neighborhood for clinical placements in community-based care? Why not collaborate with clinical agencies near CCP to meet the nursing needs in the 19130 zip code, where the college is located? Because the Kellogg project had been so successful, faculty were willing to take a chance on the 19130 Zip Code Project.

The faculty arranged community-based clinical experiences for nursing students in the neighborhood surrounding CCP. This neighborhood, where northern Center City meets North Philadelphia, would be defined by the borders of the 19130 zip code. Although CCP sits in the middle of the zip code, faculty knew little about community-based health care services in the community. The next step was to get to know the neighborhood.

In early 1995, with a 2-year grant from the Independence Foundation, the nursing faculty defined the initial Zip Code Project as serving three purposes: to develop an understanding of the characteristics and health resources in the community; to provide nursing faculty and students with the skills to conduct a community assessment; and to develop links with local community-based health care agencies (Blair, Dennehy, & White, 2005; Boyer, 1990). That spring, nursing students set out in groups of two or three, walking or driving, to complete the neighborhood needs assessment. They crisscrossed the neighborhoods within the zip code, visiting all of the agencies that offered health services, from Head Start programs to local churches. They met with each agency, asking questions, looking for unmet needs, writing profiles of local agencies, describing the health services that were being provided, and filling in survey forms.

In doing the assessment, students made a number of discoveries. In terms of shaping the Zip Code Project, two of their findings were significant: (a) The most vulnerable populations in the area were older adults and children in preschool or in grades K-5 in the public schools; and (b) the local agencies providing health care services to these groups were stretched to capacity. So faculty decided that rather than create any new services, the Zip Code Project would help local agencies expand or enhance delivery of the health care services they were already providing (Hansen-Turton & Miller, 2006).

As a result of this first community assessment, the project is now operating in more than 18 agencies throughout the neighborhood, including Head Start programs, senior citizen housing complexes, and public schools (Hansen-Turton & Miller, 2006). Since the first neighborhood assessment in 1996, each class of nursing students has updated and expanded the neighborhood assessment.

PREPARING STUDENTS FOR THE 19130
ZIP CODE PROJECT CLINICAL EXPERIENCE

Since 1996, the Zip Code Project has been integrated into the associate's degree nursing program, with all students having a project clinical experience in their second year. In the first year of the nursing program, students concentrate on medical–surgical care, learning the basics of the profession and having clinical experiences in acute care settings. To prepare them to make the most of their Zip Code Project clinical experience in the second year, students are introduced to concepts of population-based care, epidemiology, social determinants of health, and the differences and similarities between acute care and community-based care (Fiandt et al. 2004; Hayes, Miller, Miller, & Plowfield, 2009; Resick & Leonardo, 2009).

The key exercise for first-year students is assessing the neighborhood they know best—their own. Students identify where the pharmacies, clinics, physicians' offices, schools, parks, and grocery stores are located. Preparing students to complete the neighborhood assessment includes teaching them how to identify and connect with a key informant in their own neighborhood, a block captain, a neighborhood watch member, or someone else who knows the neighborhood very well. In small group discussions throughout the first year of nursing studies, faculty develop students' awareness of their own neighborhoods, talk about factors that contribute to a neighborhood's health, and consider what community residents need in order to be healthy.

In the second year of the nursing program, students repeat the community assessment assignment in the 19130 zip code. This time, they assess the neighborhood around the agency where they will have a community-based clinical experience. A two-student pair is assigned to an agency and spends 2 days each week for 6 weeks in that agency under the supervision of a master's-prepared nursing faculty member. Faculty work closely with each agency to collaborate on determining needs so they can set broad objectives for students. A typical broad objective might be to develop knowledge and skills in using a collaborative approach to assessment by working with peers, nursing faculty, community representatives, individuals, and families in the community. Objectives are broad enough for the students to talk with the agency staff to determine its needs and then create activities to meet those needs. At the same time, faculty allow students latitude in which to develop their own distinct activities for addressing the agency's health promotion and disease prevention needs.

However, the first time students go to a local agency to begin their clinical experience, they are nervous and unsure what to do. Even the community assessment activity seems unstructured. At first, everything seems ambiguous because they have just finished two semesters in acute care, where they have become accustomed to the clarity and structure of the acute care experience. But with faculty guidance, they work through the ambiguity, determine the agency's needs, and design activities to meet those needs. At the end of the experience, students are proud of their ability to deal with ambiguity. Self-confidence is a striking outcome of the students' community-based experiences, and it reflects the faculty's willingness to guide the students through the process of discovering ways to use their skills and knowledge to meet agency needs. Giving students such leeway in community-based care, however, can be difficult for some faculty, especially for those accustomed to providing the kind of close supervision required in acute care.

In both the first and second years of the nursing program, faculty continually stress the linkages between acute and community-based care. First and foremost, faculty note that every acute care client came from a community and will return to a community. Faculty encourage students in acute care to consider the community that the client is returning to: How many steps are in the home; how can the client get from his home to the pharmacy, physician, or food store; what support system does the client have in the community; and what does the client need to attend to his basic activities of daily living?

Faculty say that what they have learned by leading students in community-based experiences in the Zip Code Project has changed the way they teach. To describe their new role, faculty use the shorthand phrase, "No longer a sage from the stage but a guide from the side," meaning that they give directions, but they don't tell their students exactly what to do every step of the way. They allow and encourage students to find their own way. One result is a change in students' critical thinking skills, including challenging assumptions, reflecting, and understanding context. Faculty have found that the Zip Code Project service-learning activities facilitate the development of these essential skills (Fiandt et al., 2004; Tansey, 1999). Working in groups, students participate in discovery learning and focused inquiry. They challenge assumptions about how individuals and families access health care in the community and how and why families make decisions about using or not using specific neighborhood resources. Students report that their Zip Code Project experiences help them develop new skills including increased cultural sensitivity, the ability to cope with ambiguity, and enhanced critical thinking (Astin & Sax, 1998; Sedlak, Doheny, Panthofer, & Anaya, 2003; Strange, 2004).

PROVIDING HEALTH PROMOTION AND DISEASE PREVENTION SERVICES IN OUR COMMUNITY

Surrounding CCP's main campus in urban Philadelphia, the 19130 zip code community is distinguished by its racial and economic diversity. The community comprises approximately 50% White, 25% African American, 12% Asian, and 12% Hispanic residents. Living standards vary considerably; the average home price is $335,000, but 26% of the population lives below the federal poverty level. The 19130 zip code is experiencing economic and demographic change, with pockets of gentrification resulting in a decrease in minority and vulnerable populations since the Zip Code Project began.

As a result, nursing faculty in the project have begun to extend services into an adjacent zip code in North Philadelphia that has a very large minority population and is a medically underserved area.

All four courses in the nursing program curriculum address concepts of community-based care, cultural competence, and interdisciplinary health care, with students learning about community needs through assignments such as interviews of elderly community members (Thompson & Bucher, 2013). Examples of learning activities are provided in the following lists:

Nursing 101 (freshman/first nursing course, fall semester)

- Course term paper: Health Promotion of a Client in a Community Setting
- Seminar: Introduction to Community Assessment: Windshield Neighborhood Survey
- Seminar: Well-Elder Experience: Interview of an Elderly Person in the Community Who Lives Independently: Healthy Aging

Nursing 132 (freshman/second nursing course, spring semester)

- Course term paper: Promoting Health for the Client at Risk
- Seminar: Cultural Traditions—Lessons From Our Diverse Nursing Students

Nursing 231 (senior/third nursing course, fall semester)

- Course term paper: Community Resources for a Family Experiencing a Chronic Illness of One of Their Members
- Clinical Experience: 19130 Zip Code Project community assessment of neighborhood around assigned agency (50% of student body), including health teaching experiences in collaboration with agency staff based on a needs assessment in community agency, health surveillance activities, and collecting and recording service data on a web-based data tool
- Seminar: Family Systems

Nursing 232 (senior/fourth and final nursing course, spring semester)

- Course term paper: Philosophy of Nursing
- Clinical Experience: 19130 Zip Code Project community assessment of neighborhood around assigned agency (50% of student body), including health teaching experiences in collaboration with agency staff based on a needs assessment in community agency, health surveillance activities, and collecting and recording service data on a web-based data tool
- Seminar: Caring for HIV Clients in the Community

Direct client health promotion and disease prevention services are provided through the 19130 Zip Code Project. These services are provided by second-year nursing students under the supervision of nursing faculty based on the service-learning model (Hayes, Miller, Miller, & Plowfield, 2009). Services are provided at established community agencies such as schools and senior housing and are determined in collaboration with agency staff based on the agency's mission and needs.

Community agencies that serve vulnerable populations, including Head Start and preschool programs, public and parochial schools (K–12), senior citizen housing, and senior day care facilities, collaborate with nursing faculty and students to identify mission-based goals and activities that meet agency and student needs (Hayes, Miller, Miller, & Plowfield, 2009; Thompson & Bucher, 2013). During the 2013 calendar year, approximately 8,700 people were served, primarily in groups. (This total may include a duplicated count since, for privacy reasons, personal information is not collected from clients.) The majority of clients (70%) served were African American children (preschool through high school).

A total of 400 group health promotion and disease prevention programs were offered in 2013. The most common services provided were medication management and reconciliation/side effects, nutrition education, diabetic care education, exercise/fitness, hypertension education, child safety education, and cardiovascular education. Other prevalent group education activities included first aid, substance abuse, immunization, home safety, infection prevention, HIV/sexually transmitted infection (STI) prevention, mental/emotional health, and stress management. Prevalent surveillance services included blood pressure monitoring; height and weight measurement; vision, hearing, and temperature screening; glucose monitoring; developmental scale assessments; and head lice screening. All abnormal screenings were referred to an appropriate resource, most frequently a primary health care provider. The most prevalent reasons for referral were blood pressure, immunization, vision, hearing, and asthma. In calendar year 2013, the prevalent health promotion and education activities were medication management, nutrition, diabetic care, cardiovascular care, hypertension, exercise/fitness, and child safety.

Following each day of service, students use a web-based tool to record data about the clients they served and the services they provided. (See "The Zip Code Project Data Collection Tool: An Example of Undergraduate Postclinical Documentation" in Chapter 13 for more about this tool.) They also submit qualitative data about their perceptions of the experience. Data reports were collated, analyzed, and reviewed for six participating National Nursing Centers Consortium (NNCC) wellness centers: CCP, DeSales University, Georgia State University, LaSalle University, Temple University, and York University. Students enter data at the end of each clinical day, learning the value of reporting on types and patterns of services provided and clients served. Each school of nursing has the opportunity to preview the tool annually and suggest revisions according to their needs. Six-month and annual data reports are provided to each school of nursing. Faculty draw on these aggregate data to illustrate the value of service-learning experiences when planning the curriculum, developing grants, and negotiating with prospective community agency partners (Hazelhurst, McBurnie, Mularski, Puro, & Chauvie, 2012; Resick, Hayes, Leonardo, & Plowfield, 2009).

Direct supervision at community sites is provided by master's-prepared nursing faculty as part of their teaching assignment. The nursing faculty are experienced, respected in the community, and excellent at developing and maintaining successful relationships with community partners, which results in excellent learning experiences for students and the provision of needed wellness services for vulnerable populations in the community. Faculty collaborate with agency staff to meet the agency's needs (e.g., street safety education in preschools, medication interaction education in senior housing, hearing screening in schools; Fiandt et al., 2004). Services are determined in collaboration with agency staff based on the agency's mission and needs.

To ensure that faculty and students are prepared to provide community-based care, CCP contracted with NNCC to provide consultation and expertise in curriculum development and training for nursing students and faculty regarding social determinants of health. NNCC staff have provided training workshops to increase the capacity of nursing faculty and students to assess and address health disparities and social determinants of health. Examples of workshop topics include the landscape of health in Philadelphia, policy and the changing landscape of health care in the United States, and nurse-managed community health centers. In addition, the annual Student Development Day has been refocused to provide student and faculty development in community-based care, including health care policy.

SUSTAINABILITY AND REPLICABILITY

Faculty designed the 19130 Zip Code Project in 1996 to provide health promotion and disease prevention services to the community and to prepare nursing students for postgraduation employment in a changing health care system. At the time, hospital-based health care dominated nursing education and the field of nursing. Faculty hoped to better prepare nursing graduates for employment in other settings by integrating community-based care into the curriculum. Faculty were also motivated by growing public concerns about the need for health promotion and disease prevention services for vulnerable populations. Then as now, CCP's mission included serving the community, and in the mid-1990s, the national movement to increase community-based health care was growing.

Driven by these factors, faculty revised the nursing curriculum to better serve the community and the nursing students. By replacing hospital-based clinical experiences with community-based care, faculty responded to the community's changing needs while enhancing students' knowledge, skills, and employment opportunities (American Association of Colleges of Nursing, 1999; Boyer, 1990). Service learning in the 19130 Zip Code Project prepares nursing students to become informed and concerned citizens who can meet the changing needs of their profession and their diverse community. Faculty are intent on helping students and other faculty recognize the value of service to the local community and the need to engage in scholarship and evidence-based approaches to population-based care (Fiandt et al., 2004).

More than 1,800 nursing students have participated in the 19130 Zip Code Project since the mid-1990s. These students have gained valuable preparation for community-based care opportunities, which have grown to exceed career opportunities in hospitals. Having developed a broad range of skills, nursing graduates are well prepared for these positions. In addition, they have developed a clear understanding of community while learning to value diversity and collaboration on behalf of vulnerable populations. In recent years, over 10 alumni have earned graduate degrees in community nursing and are now serving the community in schools and agencies that serve vulnerable and minority populations (Strange, 2004).

In addition to benefiting students and community agencies, the 19130 Zip Code Project supports CCP's mission of community engagement—and provides evidence of that support to the citizens of Philadelphia. Through community-based service learning, the nursing program embodies the values of diversity and engagement that are necessary to build healthy communities and a healthy workforce (Hayes, Miller, Miller, & Plowfield, 2009).

The 19130 Zip Code Project is fully integrated into the nursing curriculum through pre- and postservice activities. All four courses in the nursing curriculum address concepts of community-based care, cultural competence, and interdisciplinary health care, with students learning about community needs through assignments such as interviews of elderly community members. Before beginning their service-learning experiences, students complete an analysis of socioeconomic and cultural aspects of the neighborhood using Internet resources and direct observation.

Through their service-learning experiences, students gain broader perspectives of their clients' lives. They learn to consider home and community environments when planning client care, deciding whether to discharge clients from the hospital, teaching clients about healthy practices, or helping them access health resources in their communities. In the process, they address community needs and build excitement about giving back to their community. Even graduates who go on to work in hospital settings value the skills and enhanced understanding of their clients' lives that they develop through the service-learning experience (Astin & Sax, 1998; Strange, 2004).

The project receives significant support from the Independence Foundation, a private, nonprofit philanthropic organization that serves Philadelphia and surrounding counties. The foundation provides CCP with an annual grant of about $15,000 to purchase supplies such as blood pressure equipment, smoking cessation materials, nutrition teaching aids, child safety coloring books, toothbrushes, and personal hygiene items.

The 19130 Zip Code Project is a well-established, stable program with strong community partners and faculty leadership. The client services provided to vulnerable, underserved clients in the 19130 Zip Code Project at CCP are health promotion and disease prevention services, based on the service-learning model; provided by second-year nursing students under the supervision of nursing faculty; provided at established community agencies such as schools and senior housing; and determined in collaboration with agency staff based on the agency's mission and needs (Hayes, Miller, Miller, & Plowfield, 2009).

In early 1995, with a 2-year grant from the Independence Foundation, the nursing faculty defined the initial Zip Code Project as serving three purposes: to develop an understanding of the characteristics and health resources in the community; to provide nursing faculty and students with the skills to conduct a community assessment; and to develop links with local community-based health care agencies. These purposes have guided the project over the ensuing years and serve as the foundation for future development.

REFERENCES

American Association of Colleges of Nursing. (1999). *Defining scholarship for the discipline of nursing.* Washington, DC: American Association of Colleges of Nursing. Retrieved from http://www.aacn.nche.edu/publications/position/defining-scholarship

Astin, L., & Sax, A. (1998). How undergraduates are affected by service participation. *Journal of College Student Development, 39*(3), 251–263.

Blair, K. A., Dennehy, P., & White, P. (2005). *Nurse practitioner faculty practice: An expectation of professionalism.* Washington, DC: National Organization of Nurse Practitioner Faculties. Retrieved from http://www.nonpf.org/resource/resmgr/imported/FPStatement2005Final.pdf

Boyer, E. L. (1990). *Scholarship reconsidered: Priorities of the professoriate.* Princeton, NJ: The Carnegie Foundation for the Advancement of Teaching.

Fiandt, K., Barr, K., Hille, G., Pelish, P., Pozehl, B., Hulme, P., . . . Burge, S. (2004). Identifying clinical scholarship faculty guidelines for faculty practice. *Journal of Professional Nursing, 20*(3), 147–155.

Hansen-Turton, T., & Miller, M. E. (2006). Nurses and nurse-managed health centers fill health care gaps. *The Pennsylvania Nurse, 61*(2), 18.

Hayes, E., Miller, J., Miller, M. E., & Plowfield, L. (2009). Community service and learning and student engagement. In T. Hansen-Turton, M. E. T. Miller, & P. A. Greiner (Eds.), *Nurse-managed wellness centers: Developing and maintaining your center* (pp. 87–103). New York, NY: Springer Publishing.

Hazelhurst, B., McBurnie, M. A., Mularski, R. A., Puro, J. E., & Chauvie, S. L. (2012). Automating care quality measurement with health information technology. *The American Journal of Managed Care, 18*(6), 312–319.

Kinsey, K., & Miller, M. E. (2012). The nursing center: A model for nursing practice in the community. In M. Stanhope & J. Lancaster (Eds.), *Public health nursing: Population centered health care in the community* (pp. 461–482). Maryland Heights: MO: Elsevier.

Resick, L. K., Hayes, E., Leonardo, M. E., & Plowfield, L. (2009). Documenting outcomes. In T. Hansen-Turton, M. E. T. Miller, & P. A. Greiner (Eds.), *Nurse-managed wellness centers: Developing and maintaining your center* (pp. 113–118). New York, NY: Springer Publishing.

Resick, L. K., & Leonardo, M. E. (2009). Application of the Boyer model of scholarship in nurse-managed wellness centers. In T. Hansen-Turton, M. E. T. Miller, & P. A. Greiner (Eds.), *Nurse-managed wellness centers: Developing and maintaining your center* (pp. 13–18). New York, NY: Springer Publishing.

Sedlak, C. A., Doheny, M. O., Panthofer, N., & Anaya, E. (2003). Critical thinking in students' service-learning experiences. *College Teaching, 51,* 99–103. doi:10.1080/87567550309596420

Strange, A. (2004). Long-term academic benefits of service-learning: When and where do they manifest themselves? *College Student Journal, 38*(2), 257–261.

Tansey, E. M. (1999). The nursing wellness center: A win-win situation for faculty. *Association of Black Nursing Faculty Journal, 10*(2), 50–51.

Thompson, C. W., & Bucher, J. A. (2013). Meeting baccalaureate public/community health nursing education competencies in nurse-managed wellness centers. *Journal of Professional Nursing, 29*(3), 155–162. doi:10.1016/j.profnurs.2012.04.017

Nurse-Managed Health Centers and Policies for the Future

Frances Hughes

For too long, nurses have been constrained in their practices by a range of legislative, administrative, funding, policy, custom, and practice barriers. Optimizing nurses' ability to work to their full, regulated scope of practice will increase flexible service delivery options and enhance options for consumers. Registered nurses working to full scope and nurse practitioners (NPs) are well placed to not only deliver safe, affordable, and accessible health care but also be the leaders and the main providers of care and services.

Expanding nurse-managed services is vital to meeting the increasing demands for services from our populations. Throughout the world, we are tackling the same issues of increased costs for medical care and treatments, health workforce constraints, the increasing burden of chronic disease, increasing consumer expectations, and population growth and aging. This means that what we have and do today must and has to change; the status quo in health care provision is not an option.

Health care has to adopt new ways of providing patient-centered care. Maximizing nurses' capacity to lead service is not only a safe, economic option; it also produces comparable or better health outcomes.

Nurse-managed services are already operating, but expansion and sustainable development are what we now need to ensure that all members of our populations have the ability to access them. We already have nurse-managed services in hospitals and communities, but new partnership models are needed to move them into areas that can not only address acute and primary care but also support consumers in improving their social determinants of health, such as mental health and addictions. Nurse-managed service can not only address the presenting problems with therapies and conventional treatments but also broker and coordinate services with consumers across the divides of education, social service, and employers. This is truly the added value of nurse-managed care—it brings the full scope of nursing in its entirety to benefit the consumer and the community.

CHAPTER 15

Workforce Trends and the Growth of the Advanced Practice Nurse Role

Sarah Hexem, Brian Valdez, and Jamie L. Ware

It is no secret that health care in the United States is undergoing dramatic change. Much of that change is based around an emerging culture of health rooted in preventive primary care and a corresponding shift in the types of providers called upon to deliver that care. This chapter reviews the policy climate around the increasing reliance on nurse practitioners (NPs) and outlines current strategies to address the demand for growth in the NP workforce. The chapter begins by situating the developing NP workforce within the culture of health and presents the NP as responsive to the emerging demand for affordable, high-quality preventive and primary care. Next, it reports current NP workforce data. Finally, it reviews provisions of the Patient Protection and Affordable Care Act (ACA) that are dedicated to workforce development and describes agency actions to advance their implementation.

THE NP IN PRIMARY CARE: LOOKING AHEAD

"As the demand for adult primary care explodes, the capacity to provide that care is shrinking," Thomas Bodenheimer and Mark Smith explain in the November 2013 issue of *Health Affairs* (Bodenheimer & Smith, 2013). At least 30 million individuals will obtain health insurance through the ACA (Congressional Budget Office, 2012). More than 8 million individuals purchased care during the inaugural open enrollment period for the health insurance marketplaces (U.S. Department of Health and Human Services [DHHS], 2014). Moreover, as of March 2014, an additional 4.8 million had obtained coverage through state Medicaid and the Children's Health Insurance Program (CHIP), another 3 million individuals under age 26 were covered under their parents' plans, and approximately 5 million people had purchased other insurance coverage. As new enrollees establish primary care homes, the burden on the primary care workforce is likely to increase dramatically. A study conducted 2 years after the state expanded its public coverage found that only 52% of internists in Massachusetts were accepting new patients and one third of family physicians no longer were (Massachusetts Medical Society, 2008). In an MSNBC article entitled "Millions Are About to Get Health Insurance. Will They Get Care?" Geoffrey Cowley (2013) writes, "If a malfunctioning website can nearly derail health care reform, imagine the fallout when people with brand-new insurance policies discover they can't get routine care."

In November 2013, the Health Resources and Services Administration's (HRSA's) National Center for Health Workforce Analysis released new data projecting the anticipated shortage of primary care providers (PCPs). The projected shortage is largely the result of an aging population, but current utilization patterns exacerbate the problem. "Without changes to how primary care is delivered, the growth in primary care physician supply will not be adequate to meet demand in 2020" (HRSA, 2013, p. 2). Other projections published by the Association of American Medical Colleges (AAMC) predict a shortage of 130,600 physicians by 2025, which includes a shortage of 65,800 primary care physicians (AAMC, 2010). And although new programs and media attention appear to have prompted some renewed interest in primary care medicine, data still show that American medical schools are not graduating enough doctors to meet this need (Jolly, Erikson, & Garrison, 2013), and the access problems are about more than just the numbers. As of January 2014, HRSA had designated 5,991 primary care Health Professional Shortage Areas, reflecting nearly 60 million individuals' limited access to care (HRSA, 2014). According to the Robert Wood Johnson Foundation (2012), NPs are also the PCPs most likely to be working in rural or remote areas.

Meanwhile, the primary care NP workforce is expanding at significantly higher rates. HRSA's 2013 projections predicted an increase of 30%, from 55,400 in 2010 to 72,100 by 2020, as compared with an 8% increase in primary care physicians (HRSA, 2013, pp. 14, 16). The U.S. Government Accountability Office reported in 2008 that compared with physicians, dentists, and physician assistants (PAs), NPs are the fastest growing segment of PCPs in the country. Not surprisingly, health care policy makers are increasingly looking to them to assume a greater role in primary care. Since its 2011 future of nursing report, the Institute of Medicine (IOM) has been calling on NPs "to fulfill and expand their potential as primary care providers across practice settings based on their education and competency" (IOM, 2011, p. 1). Following suit, the National Governor's Association, the National Institute for Health Care Reform, and the National Center for Health Workforce Analysis all assert that increasing NP primary care can alleviate pressure on the primary care workforce (DHHS, 2012; National Governors Association, 2012; Yee, 2013).

Moreover, as policy makers increasingly turn to more efficient models of health care (NPs, for example), a RAND study projected that greater use of the nurse-managed health clinic (NMHC) model could address the increased demand for primary care (Auerbach et al., 2013), given that they are primarily managed by NPs. When discussing the role of NMHCs, the IOM report says, "Nurse-managed health clinics offer opportunities to expand access; provide quality, evidence-based care; and improve outcomes for individuals who may not otherwise receive needed care" (IOM, 2011, p. c4).

THE NP WORKFORCE BY THE NUMBERS

According to HRSA's 2012 National Sample Survey of Nurse Practitioners, there were an estimated 154,000 NPs in the United States (see Figure 15.1; HRSA, 2014). More than 85% practiced in positions that require an NP

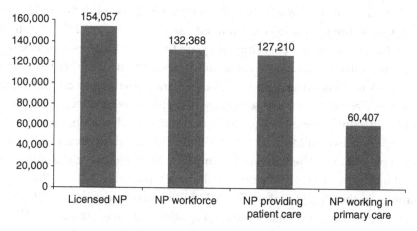

Figure 15.1 Estimated nurse practitioner supply, 2012 (HRSA, 2014).
HRSA, Health Resources and Services Administration; NP, nurse practitioner.

credential. Approximately 96% of these NPs provided patient care, and about half (60,407) worked in primary care. Of the total NP workforce, 94% had graduate degrees.

As the number of NPs has grown, so has the number of patients receiving NP care. According to a 2010 study by the American Academy of Nurse Practitioners, 81% of Americans have seen, or know someone close to them who has seen, an NP for their health care (Aleshire, Wheeler, & Prevost, 2012). A similar study showed that from 1998 to 2010, the proportion of Medicare patients for whom NPs billed increased 9.5% in outpatient settings (Kuo, Loresto, Rounds, & Goodwin, 2013). Following this trend, from 2006 to 2010, the percentage of patients with PCPs who were NPs increased significantly across all states. Notably, Kuo and colleagues documented a strong association between states with restrictions on NP practice and the percentage of patients with NP PCPs.

RAND projects that the number of trained NPs will increase by 94% by the year 2025 (from 128,000 in 2008 to 244,000; Auerbach, 2012). The Bureau of Labor Statistics (2014) likewise predicts an increase in the supply of advanced practice nurses (APNs, including nurse anesthetists and nurse midwives as well as NPs) of 31% between 2012 and 2022. However, realization of these numbers depends in part on the availability of workforce education and training. The American Association of Colleges of Nursing (AACN) reports that in 2012, nursing schools turned down 79,659 qualified applicants from baccalaureate and graduate nursing programs because of insufficient number of faculty, clinical sites, classroom space, and clinical preceptors, as well as budget constraints (Fang, Li, & Bednash, 2013). Of the nursing schools that responded to AACN's *2012–2013 Enrollment and Graduations in Baccalaureate and Graduate Programs in Nursing* report, nearly two thirds cited faculty shortages as the reason for their limited capacity (Rosseter, 2014). Cultivating APN educators and ensuring adequate financing for nursing workforce programs will be critical to the continuing development of the NP workforce.

Lack of diversity among NPs also demands attention as current trends continue. Recent years have seen increased efforts toward recruiting APNs from culturally diverse backgrounds, and nurse academics have identified the importance of building an NP workforce that can deliver culturally competent patient care (The Nursing Community, 2008). However, the ethnic and racial makeup of the NP workforce still differs dramatically from the demographics in the United States. The 2012 HRSA survey depicts an NP workforce that is "largely homogeneous in gender and race/ethnicity" (HRSA, 2014, p. 4). Only 3% of respondents identified as Hispanic/Latino and 5% as Black (non-Hispanic), and 6% fell within "other non-Hispanic groups" (HRSA, 2014, p. 4). Just 7% of the NP workforce was male.

FEDERAL POLICIES TO ADVANCE THE ADVANCED PRACTICE NURSING WORKFORCE

Responding to the shortage of health providers delivering primary and preventive care, the federal government is actively developing the nursing workforce. Historically, this was accomplished through nursing workforce development programs (Title VIII of the Public Health Service Act, 42 U.S.C. 296 et seq.), primarily federal grants, loans, and scholarships to nursing students and educational institutions. The ACA expanded this support by investing in new programs and reauthorizing and extending prior programs that were first enacted in Title VIII.

50 Years of Nursing Workforce Development

In 2014, the Nursing Workforce Development programs established under Title VIII celebrate their 50th year (www.thenursingcommunity.org). HRSA, a part of DHHS, administers the programs that develop nursing recruitment, education, practice, and retention at all levels. Between 2006 and 2012, over 450,000 nurses and nursing students received Title VIII program funding. Federal funds also supported health care facilities and nursing schools.

Expanding Workforce Development Through the ACA

Through the ACA, Congress sought to remedy the twin problems of the current shortage of nurses and the lack of institutional capacity to train them. New and expanded funding programs provide additional financial aid to nursing students and offer loans to nursing schools to enable them to increase their capacity (see Figure 15.2). The ACA also invests in primary care programs, where nurses play a vital role. The full impact of the ACA on the nursing workforce is yet to be seen, particularly as more states elect to expand Medicaid and thereby see more demand for accessible, affordable, high-quality care. However, this section provides a brief overview of current nursing workforce development programs established by the ACA. Through these and other initiatives, the ACA is slated to add 600 new NPs and nurse midwives to the workforce by 2015 (White House, n.d.).

Graduate Nursing Education Demonstration Program

Section 5509 of the ACA (2010c) requires the secretary to establish a 4-year graduate nurse education demonstration program under Medicare. The ACA authorizes up to $50 million per year to reimburse five hospitals for clinical

2010—On March 23, 2010, President Obama signed into law the Patient Protection and Affordable Care Act (P.L. 111–148). This health care reform legislation expanded certain provisions of the Title VIII programs, including increasing aggregate loan levels for the Nursing Student Loan Program from $13,000 to $17,000, and expanding the educational loan repayment amount from $30,000 to $35,500 for the Nurse Faculty Loan Program.

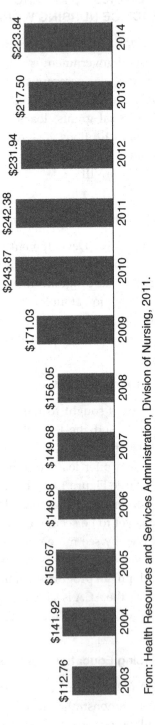

Year	Amount
2003	$112.76
2004	$141.92
2005	$150.67
2006	$149.68
2007	$149.68
2008	$156.05
2009	$171.03
2010	$243.87
2011	$242.38
2012	$231.94
2013	$217.50
2014	$223.84

From: Health Resources and Services Administration, Division of Nursing, 2011.

Figure 15.2 Funding for the Title VIII Workforce Development Program.

training expenses incurred in the education of NPs and other APNs. Only those expenses that exceed the hospitals' normal projected expenditures will be reimbursed, which provides an incentive for the hospitals to expand their APN clinical training programs. The program also requires that 50% of all clinical training opportunities occur in nonhospital, community-based settings. However, the provision does allow hospitals in rural or medically underserved areas to waive the community-based care setting requirement. On July 30, 2012, the Center for Medicare & Medicaid Innovation announced awards to the following demonstration sites: the Hospital of the University of Pennsylvania (Philadelphia, PA), Duke University Hospital (Durham, NC), Scottsdale Healthcare Medical Center (Scottsdale, AZ), Rush University Medical Center (Chicago, IL), and Memorial Hermann-Texas Medical Center Hospital (Houston, TX). Demonstrations are slated to run for 4 years, at which point the secretary will report on the program's success and number of APNs prepared.

NP Training in FQHCs and NMHCs

Section 5316 of the ACA (2010b) authorizes the secretary to establish a training demonstration program to train NPs for careers as PCPs in federally qualified health centers (FQHCs) and NMHCs. Three-year grants were to be awarded to employ and provide 1 year of training to qualifying family NPs who had graduated from an NP program. Only FQHCs and NMHCs would have been eligible for the incentives, and grants were limited to $600,000 each year. Priority was to be given to those FQHCs or NMHCs that demonstrated sufficient infrastructure and capacity to train at least three NPs per year; provided NPs with specialty rotations; provided sessions on high-volume, high-risk health problems; and collaborated with other safety-net providers. However, the program has yet to be funded.

Section 330 of the Public Health Service Act (42 USCS § 254b, 2014) provides financial assistance and other benefits, including increased Medicare and Medicaid reimbursement, to qualifying community health centers that provide primary care in medically underserved areas. To qualify, health centers must have certain elements, including a governing board of directors with more than 50% individuals from the patient community to be served.

Safety-net health centers affiliated with academic nursing institutions frequently cannot meet the FQHC board requirement, which deprives them of the opportunity to access the related benefits. The ACA addresses this issue by separately authorizing up to $50 million for an NMHC grant program. Section 5208 (ACA, 2010a) authorizes funds to develop and operate

NMHCs that provide comprehensive primary health care services without regard to patient income or insurance status for the duration of the grant. The inclusion of this provision in the ACA addresses NMHCs' important and unique role in providing high-need communities with high-quality care while also functioning as clinical training sites. Ten NMHCs were funded in 2010 by the NMHC grant program, but Congress has not since appropriated any additional funding, and NMHCs continue to struggle with inadequate funding.

In 2012, the National Nursing Centers Consortium (NNCC) conducted a survey of its members to measure their contributions to health professions education. Ninety-six percent of respondents reported that their NMHCs served as training sites for students in nursing and other health professions programs. Twenty-eight NMHCs in a mix of urban, rural, and suburban communities reported providing educational opportunities for nearly 1,500 students (www.nncc.us/site). The average number of students educated by the NMHC grant-funded clinics was 80, while the clinics participating in the 2012 survey reported educating an average of 55 students. These results connect increased funding with the ability of NMHCs to offer education opportunities that advance workforce development (see Figure 15.3).

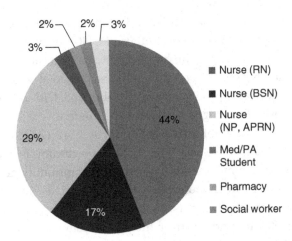

Figure 15.3 Types of students who complete clinical rotations in nurse-managed health clinics.

APRN, advanced practice registered nurse; BSN, bachelor of science in nursing; NP, nurse practitioner; PA, physician assistant.

U.S. Public Health Sciences Track

Section 5315 of the ACA authorizes the establishment of a U.S. Public Health Sciences Track. The secretary shall select sites with authority to grant advanced graduate degrees that emphasize team-based service, public health, epidemiology, and emergency preparedness and response. The statute requires that the track be organized such that no fewer than 250 nursing students and 100 PAs or NPs graduate annually. Selected students shall be awarded annual tuition and stipends through up to 4 years of schooling, in return for a promise to work for a period of time in the Commissioned Corps of the Public Health Service after completion of the track. Beginning with fiscal year 2010, the secretary shall transfer from the Public Health and Social Services Emergency Fund such sums as may be necessary to carry out this section.

Nurse and Faculty Loan Program

Section 5311 expands the amount of annual federal loans available under the School of Nursing Student Loan Fund from $30,000 to $35,000 (adjusted for cost of attendance after 2011). The section also creates an Eligible Individual Loan Repayment program, which provides educational loan repayment for individuals who agree to serve as full-time faculty at an accredited school of nursing for a total aggregate of 4 years out of a 6-year period.

Bureau of Health Workforce

In May 2014, HRSA announced that it would be combining workforce programs from the Bureau of Clinician Recruitment and Services and the Bureau of Health Professions to form a new Bureau of Health Workforce. The new bureau will administer many of the programs described earlier as well as collect and analyze health workforce data. The bureau intends to prepare the health care workforce "to improve the public health by expanding access to quality health services and working to achieve health equity."

CONCLUSION

Although much remains to be seen, it is certain that the role of the NP will continue to be important in the evolving landscape of health care in the United States.

REFERENCES

Aleshire, M. E., Wheeler, K., & Prevost, S. S. (2012). The future of nurse practitioner practice: A world of opportunity. *The Nursing Clinics of North America, 47*(2), 181–191, doi:10.1016/j.cnur.2012.04.002

Association of American Medical Colleges (AAMC). (2010). *The impact of health care reform on the future supply and demand for physicians updated projections through 2025.* Washington, DC: Association of American Medical Colleges. Retrieved from https://www.aamc.org/download/158076/data/updated_projections_through_2025.pdf

Auerbach, D. I. (2012). Will the NP workforce grow in the future? New forecasts and implications for health care delivery. *Medical Care, 50*(7), 606–610. doi:10.1097/MLR.0b013e318249d6e7

Auerbach, D. I., Chen, P. G., Friedberg, M. W., Reid, R., Lau, C., Buerhaus, P. I., & Mehrotra, A. (2013). Nurse-managed health centers and patient-centered medical homes could mitigate expected primary care physician shortage. *Health Affairs (Project Hope), 32*(11), 1933–1941. doi:10.1377/hlthaff.2013.0596

Bodenheimer, T. S., & Smith, M. D. (2013). Primary care: Proposed solutions to the physician shortage without training more physicians. *Health Affairs (Project Hope), 32*(11), 1881–1886. doi:10.1377/hlthaff.2013.0234

Bureau of Labor Statistics. (2014). *Occupational outlook handbook, 2014–15 edition, nurse anesthetists, nurse midwives, and nurse practitioners.* Washington, DC: Bureau of Labor Statistics. Retrieved from http://www.bls.gov/ooh/healthcare/nurse-anesthetists-nurse-midwives-and-nurse-practitioners.htm

Congressional Budget Office. (2012). *Estimates for the insurance coverage provisions of the Affordable Care Act updated for the recent Supreme Court decision.* Retrieved from http://www.cbo.gov/sites/default/files/cbofiles/attachments/43472-07-24-2012-CoverageEstimates.pdf

Cowley, G. (2013, December 2). Millions are about to get health insurance. Will they get care? *MSNBC.* Retrieved from http://www.msnbc.com/msnbc/doctor-gap-next-hurdle-health-care

Fang, D., Li, Y., & Bednash, G. D. (2013). *2012–2013 enrollment and graduations in baccalaureate and graduate programs in nursing.* Washington, DC: American Association of Colleges of Nursing. Retrieved from http://www.aacn.nche.edu/downloads/ids/2013/EG12.pdf

Health Resources and Services Administration (HRSA). (2013). *Projecting the supply and demand for primary care practitioners through 2020.* Retrieved from http://bhpr.hrsa.gov/healthworkforce/supplydemand/usworkforce/primarycare/projectingprimarycare.pdf

Health Resources and Services Administration (HRSA). (2014). *Highlights from the 2012 National Sample Survey of Nurse Practitioners.* Retrieved from http://bhpr.hrsa.gov/healthworkforce/supplydemand/nursing/nursepractitionersurvey/

Institute of Medicine (IOM). (2011). *The future of nursing: Leading change, advancing health.* Washington, DC: The National Academies Press.

Jolly, P., Erikson, C., & Garrison, G. (2013). U.S. graduate medical education and physician specialty choice. *Academic Medicine: Journal of the Association of American Medical Colleges, 88*(4), 468–474. doi:10.1097/ACM.0b013e318285199d

Kuo, Y.-F., Loresto, F. L., Rounds, L. R., & Goodwin, J. S. (2013). States with the least restrictive regulations experienced the largest increase in patients seen by nurse practitioners. *Health Affairs (Project Hope), 32*(7), 1236–1243. doi:10.1377/hlthaff.2013.0072

Massachusetts Medical Society. (2008). *Physician workforce study: Executive summary.* Waltham, MA: Massachusetts Medical Society. Retrieved from http://media.wickedlocal.com/pdf/MMS_Executive_Summary.pdf

National Governors Association. (2012). *The role of nurse practitioners in meeting increasing demand for primary care.* Washington, DC: National Governors Association. Retrieved from http://www.nga.org/cms/home/nga-center-for-best-practices/center-publications/page-health-publications/col2-content/main-content-list/the-role-of-nurse-practitioners.html

Nursing Community. (2008). *Consensus document: Reauthorization priorities for Title VIII, Public Health Service Act (42 U.S.C. 296 et seq.).* Retrieved from http://www.aacn.org/WD/Practice/Docs/PublicPolicy/Nursing_Consensus_Document.pdf

Patient Protection and Affordable Care Act (ACA), Pub. L. No. 111-148, § 5208, 612 Stat. 124. (2010a).

Patient Protection and Affordable Care Act (ACA), Pub. L. No. 111-148, § 5316, 995 Stat. 124. (2010b).

Patient Protection and Affordable Care Act (ACA), Pub. L. No. 111-148, § 5509, 674 Stat. 124. (2010c).

Public Health Service Act, 42 USC §254(c)-1a(e). (2014).

Robert Wood Johnson Foundation. (2012). *Implementing the IOM future of nursing report-part III: How nurses are solving some of primary care's most pressing challenges.* Princeton, NJ: Robert Wood Johnson Foundation. Retrieved from http://www.rwjf.org/content/dam/files/rwjf-web-files/Resources/2/cnf20120810.pdf

Rosseter, R. J. (2014). *Nursing faculty shortage fact sheet.* Washington, DC: American Association of Colleges of Nursing. Retrieved from http://www.aacn.nche.edu/media-relations/FacultyShortageFS.pdf

Title VIII of the Public Health Service Act, 42 U.S.C. 296 et seq. (2014).

U.S. Department of Health and Human Services, Agency for Healthcare Research and Quality. (2012, January). *Primary care workforce facts and stats: Overview.* Rockville, MD: Author.

U.S. Department of Health and Human Services, Agency for Healthcare Research and Quality. (2014, October). *Primary care workforce facts and stats no. 3.* Retrieved from http://www.ahrq.gov/research/findings/factsheets/primary/pcwork3/index.html

U.S. Department of Health and Human Services (DHHS). (2014). *Enrollment in the health insurance marketplace totals over 8 million people.* Retrieved from http://www.hhs.gov/news/press/2014pres/05/20140501a.html

White House. (n.d.). *The Obama administration's record on supporting the nursing workforce.* Retrieved from http://www.whitehouse.gov/sites/default/files/docs/nurses_report.pdf

Yee, T., Boukus, E., Cross, D. & Samuel, D. (2013). *Primary care workforce shortages: Nurse practitioner scope-of-practice laws and payment policies.* (Research Brief No. 13). Washington, DC: National Institute for Health Care Reform.

CHAPTER 16

THE FUTURE OF NURSE-MANAGED CARE AND NATIONAL POLICY EFFORTS

Brian Valdez, Sarah Hexem, and Jamie M. Ware

The future of nurse-managed care in the United States changed forever in 2010. The sweeping reforms introduced by the passage of the Affordable Care Act (ACA) in March of that year gave nurse-managed health clinics (NMHCs) an unprecedented level of recognition and access to previously unavailable funding sources. Following the enactment of the law, the Institute of Medicine (IOM) released a groundbreaking report entitled *The Future of Nursing: Leading Change, Advancing Health* (2010) that called on nurses, particularly advanced practice nurses (APNs), to assume a greater role in primary care and highlighted the potential of NMHCs to deliver care to vulnerable populations. This chapter examines the impact of the ACA and the IOM report on nurse-managed care, gives an overview of what has happened since 2010, and looks at some ways these documents are expected to advance nurse-managed care in the future.

THE ACA AND ITS RELEVANCE FOR NMHCs

The passage of the ACA was a momentous occasion for NMHCs for two reasons. First, the law officially recognized NMHCs as safety-net providers by defining the term NMHC in federal law. According to Section 5208 of the ACA, an NMHC is "a nurse practice arrangement, managed by advanced practice nurses (APN), that provides primary care or wellness services to underserved or vulnerable populations and that is associated with a school, college, university or department of nursing, federally qualified health center, or independent nonprofit health or social services agency" (ACA, 2010a). The inclusion of this language in the Public Health Service Act places NMHCs on the same level as other safety-net providers like federally qualified health centers (FQHCs). The definition also opens the door for NMHCs to participate in federally funded programs and take advantage of new funding sources.

Second, the ACA created the NMHC Grant Program, a federally funded grant program specifically for NMHCs. Section 5208, cited earlier, gives the secretary of the U.S. Department of Health and Human Services (DHHS) the authority to make grants to fund the growth and development of NMHCs. It also authorizes Congress to appropriate up to $50,000,000 for the grants (2010a).

Many of the nation's NMHCs struggle financially because they are affiliated with schools of nursing and cannot qualify for the grant funds available to other safety-net providers like FQHCs and rural health clinics. The grant program was intended to solve this problem by giving NMHCs grant funds they could use to offset the cost of caring for the uninsured and stabilize the model. Although Congress has never allocated any funds to the program, in 2010, DHHS awarded $1.5 million grants to 10 of the nation's NMHCs with funds from the ACA's Prevention and Public Health Fund. Each year of the 3-year grant cycle, the grantees cared for an average of 27,000 patients, recorded over 72,000 encounters, and served as clinical placement sites for 800 health profession students (National Nursing Centers Consortium [NNCC], 2012).

In addition to the provisions that directly relate to NMHCs, the ACA has benefited the clinics in other ways. For example, Section 5316 of the Act established a 1-year demonstration project to fund residency programs for family nurse practitioners (NPs) to be educated and trained in NMHCs or FQHCs (ACA, 2010b). Section 5509 also created a 5-year graduate nurse education demonstration project (ACA, 2010c). Finally, the ACA provides funding for community health centers (CHCs) and school-based health centers, many of which are NMHCs. Support for these types of clinics has led to increased employment opportunities for APNs and other nurses. CHCs, for example, have added 3,000 nursing positions since 2009, and 800 of these have gone to APNs (White House, n.d.). Overall, the number of APNs working in CHCs has grown by 20% in the past 5 years (White House, n.d.).

In a more general way, the ACA will benefit NMHCs by increasing their numbers of insured patients. An estimated 12 million individuals were expected to gain coverage through various ACA initiatives by the end of 2014 (Congressional Budget Office, 2014). Nationally, nearly half of all NMHC patients are uninsured (IOM, 2010). Extending coverage to currently uninsured NMHC patients will increase the reimbursement revenue available to the clinics.

How It Happened

The ACA's support of NMHCs was not an accident; it was the result of a prolonged advocacy campaign that began in the mid-1990s. In the late 1980s and early 1990s, the federal government enacted a series of laws aimed at countering what was then a growing nursing shortage. This focus on building the nation's nursing workforce sparked a renewed interest in the NMHC model, which has the capacity to provide nursing students with community-based clinical experience while increasing access to care for vulnerable patients. By 1992, the Health Resources and Services Administration's (HRSA's) Division of Nursing (DoN) had funded 17 new NMHCs through its Nurse, Education, Practice, Quality and Retention grant program. The division continued its investment, and by 2000, the number of NMHCs had grown to 200 (Hansen-Turton, Miller, & Grenier, 2009). Most of the NMHCs in existence today can trace their roots back to DoN grants awarded during this time period.

Shortly after beginning operations, many of the newly funded NMHCs realized they needed a vehicle for voicing their concerns around national and state policies that they felt were unnecessarily restricting their freedom of practice and interfering with their ability to adequately care for their patients. NNCC, a 501(c)(3) nonprofit membership association representing the nation's NMHCs, was founded to fulfill this need. The organization's policy team works with policy makers at the state and national levels to address barriers to NMHC practice and secure sustainable NMHC funding.

Early on, NNCC found that very few legislators understood the NMHC model or what NPs and other APNs were capable of doing. Therefore, the organization's policy staff began by raising awareness of NMHCs and promoting the recognition of NPs in state law. One of NNCC's first policy achievements on this front was to help NPs in Pennsylvania win the right to prescribe medications. NNCC continued its advocacy around NP prescriptive authority, and today NPs can prescribe in all 50 states—Georgia became the last state to extend this privilege in 2006.

NNCC's initial strategy for raising awareness in Congress mainly involved working with key members to insert language about NMHCs into the *Congressional Record*. An early example of this language is included in the following text:

> Nurse-managed health centers are nationally recognized safety-net primary health care providers in urban and rural areas. The majority of nurse-run health centers have been established by non-profit, university-based schools of nursing to meet the needs and interests of community members and to prepare qualified graduates with the skills to work in medically underserved areas. Many of these health centers were originally funded by the U.S. Department of Health and Human Services, Health Resources and Services Administration (HRSA), Bureau of Health Professions and Division of Nursing. Critical goals for the nurse-managed primary care health centers include attaining Federally Qualified Health Center status and becoming contributing members of the Consolidated Health Centers Program….The committee encourages HRSA's Bureau of Primary Health Care to expedite FQHC certification and, where appropriate, provide 330 funding to nurse-managed health centers…previously and are currently funded by HRSA, Bureau of Health Professions, Division of Nursing….(U.S. Senate Health, Education, Labor, and Pensions Committee Report Accompanying the 2001 Health Care Safety Net Act (S. 1533)

It was through this process of working to get NMHCs cited in the *Congressional Record* that NNCC first developed a relationship with three of its biggest congressional champions: former Senators Arlen Specter (D-PA) and Daniel Inouye (D-HI) and current Republican Senator Lamar Alexander of Tennessee. During his long tenure, Senator Inouye was one of nursing's strongest supporters in the Senate. Cultivating this relationship proved critical to NNCC's efforts to get NMHC language included in the ACA.

NNCC's policy team quickly realized that focusing on scope of practice issues like prescriptive authority was not enough; they also needed to open up new sources of funding for NMHCs. Most safety-net clinics like FQHCs and rural health clinics receive federal funding in the form of grants and increased reimbursement rates. Because the majority of NMHCs are affiliated with schools of nursing, they fall under the governance authority of a university or college and cannot meet the federal requirements regarding the governance of the center. Like other safety-net providers, NMHCs see a large percentage of uninsured patients, and by the early 2000s, the inability of the clinics to access these enhanced funding sources began to pose a real threat to the model's sustainability. The DoN grants that had helped found so many NMHCs began to run out, and it became clear that unless NNCC and other advocates took steps to open up new avenues for federal support, a large percentage of the formerly DoN-funded NMHCs would close due to lack of revenue.

In 2006, NNCC and other nursing groups came together to introduce a federal bill that would solve this problem. The bill was designed to grant NMHCs seeking FQHC funding under Section 330 of the Public Health Service Act a temporary waiver of the 51% governance board requirement. With this waiver in place, NMHCs would have access to federal funding while they worked to develop governance boards that were in compliance with all federal regulations. The bill, which represented NNCC's first attempt to introduce federal legislation, did not become law. However, the group learned two important lessons during this process. The first was that in order to effectively move federal legislation, they needed a broad base of support among nursing groups and CHC advocates. Second, NNCC decided that rather than attempting to alter the existing FQHC and rural health clinic grant program, it would seek to establish a new grant program specifically for NMHCs.

Building off these lessons, NNCC began working with a core group of nursing organizations and other allies, such as the National Association of Community Health Centers, to draft and introduce the Nurse Managed Health Clinic Investment Act of 2007. This bill, which was introduced in the U.S. Senate by Senators Inouye and Alexander, sought to create a grant program solely for NMHCs. Under this legislation, NMHCs would be able to compete for federal funding without having to establish the governance board required under the FQHC regulations. Instead, they would set up community advisory boards that allowed the community to have a voice in the operation of university-affiliated NMHCs without the school of nursing having to surrender governance authority. This bill did not become law, but it did gain key cosponsors in the Senate, one of whom was Vice President Joe Biden, then a senator from Delaware.

NNCC and its nursing allies reintroduced the NMHC Investment Act in 2009. By this time, the climate in Washington had completely changed. Barack Obama had been elected president, and the Democrats had gained control of both houses of Congress. Along with reintroducing the bill in the Senate, NNCC was able to introduce a companion bill in the U.S. House of Representatives. Representative Lois Capps (D-CA 24), who is one of nursing's biggest congressional champions, was an original sponsor of the legislation. She was joined by Representative Lee Terry (R-NE 02). In part because of her important position on the House Energy and Commerce Committee, Representative Capps was able to include the NMHC bill language in the ACA legislation as it moved through the committee.

The bill in the Senate was again supported by Senators Inouye and Alexander. Senator Inouye's staff included a military nurse who worked tirelessly to move the bill forward. Through her efforts, NNCC was able to secure a meeting with staff from the office of Senator Edward Kennedy (D-MA), who was then Chairman of the Senate Committee on Health, Education, Labor, and Pensions. Senator Kennedy's staff subsequently agreed to insert the NMHC bill language into the Senate's version of the ACA legislation. With the language safely included in both the House and Senate versions, the NMHC Investment Act was all but guaranteed to become law when the ACA passed.

What's Happening Now

The inclusion of a formal NMHC definition in the ACA did place NMHCs on the same level as other safety-net providers in terms of recognition. However, it did not give the clinics access to consistent sources of federal funding. Deep partisan divisions in Washington, budget constraints, and the backlash against health care reform have made it difficult to find support for any program associated with the ACA. As a result, Congress has not appropriated any funding to the NMHC grant program. The 10 NMHC grants that were funded through the ACA's Prevention and Public Health Fund have since expired and have not been renewed. The program itself has expired and is awaiting reauthorization. NNCC is currently working with other advocates on a campaign to get the law reauthorized.

Likewise, the one-year NP education and training demonstration project created under Section 5316 of the ACA has not been renewed. Section 5509's Graduate Nurse Education demonstration project is still in the process of being completed. While a small number of NMHCs have benefited from this project, the program is hospital led. NNCC is currently partnering with the National Association of Community Health Centers to craft a new clinic-led demonstration that would place a greater emphasis on providing nursing students with education and training through community-based placements in NMHCs, FQHCs, and retail clinics.

THE IOM'S *THE FUTURE OF NURSING* REPORT
AND ITS IMPACT ON NMHCs

In the wake of the ACA's passage, the IOM, one of the most respected analytical bodies in the United States, released a landmark report, *The Future of Nursing*. The report, the product of an intense 2-year consensus study, was completed in October 2010. It contains 8 recommendations and 42 subrecommendations designed to transform nursing in a way that meets the immense health care needs of the United States and places the workforce in a position to succeed in the changing health care environment (Fairman & Okoye, 2011). A major theme of the report is that nurses, especially APNs, should be called upon to fulfill and expand their potential as primary care providers (PCPs). To ensure that this occurs, the report recommends that government administrators, legislators, third-party payers, and other stakeholders work together to remove scope of practice barriers that unnecessarily restrict the functions APNs can perform. Specifically, the report's first recommendation is that "APNs should be able to practice to the full extent of their education and training" (IOM, 2010, p. 4).

Some of the subrecommendations accompanying this overall recommendation include

- A call for policy makers to remove outdated and unnecessary restrictions on APN practice
- A call for third-party payers in fee-for-service to provide direct reimbursement to APNs
- A call for APNs to be granted clinical and admitting privileges (IOM, 2010)

Although the report's other recommendations deal with nurses of all levels, they support an expanded primary care role for APNs by calling for things like establishing APN residency programs, developing nursing curricula that emphasize the cultivation of entrepreneurial skills, and placing nurses in interdisciplinary leadership positions (IOM, 2010).

Any push toward the removal of unnecessary scope of practice barriers and a greater presence for nurses in primary care is going to benefit NMHCs. But the report also takes time to specifically highlight NMHCs and several nurse-managed practice models. The terms "nurse-managed health clinic" or "NMHC" appear over 40 times throughout the 600-page report, and on page 319, IOM states: "Nurse-managed health clinics offer opportunities to expand access; provide quality, evidence-based care; and improve outcomes for individuals who may not otherwise receive needed care" (IOM, 2010).

Along with talking generally about NMHC patient demographics, the contribution of the clinics to primary care, and their role in workforce development, the report gives examples of successful nurse-managed models of care around the country. Some of these include NMHCs serving vulnerable populations in Philadelphia, Pennsylvania, and Galveston, Texas, as well as nurse-managed programs serving the elderly and migrant farm workers (IOM, 2010).

What's Happening Now

Following its release, the report's organizers, along with nursing supporters, consumer groups, and other stakeholders, began a nationwide campaign to make certain its recommendations were fully implemented. This process is currently ongoing. Some of the principal architects of this effort, known as the Future of Nursing: Campaign for Action, include the Robert Wood Johnson Foundation, a private philanthropic foundation with a long-standing commitment to nurses, as well as AARP (Fairman & Okoye, 2011). The campaign, which is coordinated through the Center to Champion Nursing in America, envisions a health care system in which all Americans have access to high-quality care, with nurses contributing to the full extent of their capabilities. Campaign for Action chapters are active in all 50 states. NNCC is a member of the Pennsylvania chapter as well as a contributor on the campaign's national board.

Significant progress has been made in the 4 years since the report. For example, the report set goals to increase the percentage of baccalaureate or higher level nurses to 80% by 2020 and to double the number of nurses with doctorates (IOM, 2010). According to the American Association of Colleges of Nursing, enrollments for RN-to-BSN programs were up more than 22% in 2012 (Wood, 2013). There has also been a 27% increase in enrollment in Doctor of Nursing Practice programs and a 4% increase in PhD nursing programs (Wood, 2013). In the area of scope of practice reforms, statistics show that in 2013, 16 states introduced legislation to remove scope of practice barriers (Wood, 2013).

FUTURE DIRECTIONS

Although partisan politics has slowed reforms at the federal level, the ACA and *The Future of Nursing* have greatly improved the position of NMHCs and nurse-managed practice in the states. State legislators across the country are heeding the call to expand the roles of APNs and NMHCs in primary care. One indication of the move toward greater acceptance of NMHCs is the growth in the number of states that allow NPs to practice independent of physician supervision. Currently, 18 states and the District of Columbia allow NPs to practice independently. Nevada, Rhode Island, Connecticut, and Oregon are the most recent states to be added to this list—all passed legislation granting NPs full practice authority in 2013 or early 2014 (please note that these laws require nurse practitioners to meet certain requirements pertaining to things like practice, education, and experience before they can practice independently). Kentucky also recently passed a law that allows APNs with 4 or more years of practice experience to prescribe most medications without a collaborative practice agreement, although the law still requires a written agreement when prescribing certain controlled substances. NNCC expects the trend toward greater independence for APNs to increase as state policy makers look to augment the number of PCPs available to care for newly insured patients receiving coverage under the ACA's Medicaid expansion.

Another place where NNCC has seen the ACA and IOM report making an impact for NMHCs is in the area of managed care credentialing. Although NPs are legally qualified to act as PCPs in all 50 states and the District of Columbia, managed care organizations (MCOs) have traditionally been reluctant to recognize NPs and other APNs as PCPs. The refusal of many MCOs to contract with NPs is another barrier that continues to limit the reimbursement available to NMHCs. In an effort to determine the extent of the problem, NNCC conducts a biannual survey of the NP credentialing and reimbursement practices among the nation's largest health maintenance organizations (HMOs).

The most recent survey, completed in 2011, involved a total of 258 HMOs serving patients across the country. The results showed that only 75% of the HMOs surveyed permitted NPs to serve as PCPs in their provider networks, 24% indicated that they did not credential NPs as PCPs, and 1% stated that they allowed NPs to serve as PCPs only under certain circumstances (Hansen-Turton, Ware, Bond, Doria, & Cunningham, 2013). Among the different HMO types, Medicare plans were most likely to credential NPs as PCPs, while commercial plans were the least likely. The credentialing rate for Medicare plans was 83%, followed by Medicaid plans at 75% and commercial plans at 67% (Hansen-Turton et al., 2013). The survey also found that 27% of the participating health plans reimbursed NPs at the same level as physicians, 27% reported reimbursing NPs at a lower level than physicians, and 46% said that the rate at which NPs were reimbursed varied depending on the contract (Hansen-Turton et al., 2013).

While it is troubling that nearly a quarter of the nation's managed care companies still will not recognize NPs as PCPs, the survey revealed that the percentage of HMOs that credential NPs as PCPs has grown over 20% since NNCC last conducted the survey in 2009 (Hansen-Turton et al., 2013). Perhaps the biggest factor contributing to this increase is recognition on the part of managed care executives that their PCP networks are not sufficient to handle the surge in newly insured individuals that is resulting from the passage of the ACA. Another factor is the rise of the nation's 1,600 retail-based convenient care clinics. The majority of these clinics based in high-traffic retail outlets are nurse managed. The rapid expansion of the retail clinic industry has helped place added pressure on MCOs to contract with APNs as PCPs.

CONCLUSION

Although the passage of the ACA and release of the IOM report represented tremendous steps forward for the nation's NMHCs, there is more work to be done. These centers are still in need of a sustainable source of federal funding, a large percentage of managed care companies maintain policies that prevent NPs from serving as PCPs even in the face of a growing demand for primary care, and some states have begun to pass laws that limit NP scope of practice by making NPs practice as part of physician-led teams. Unless state and federal policy makers move to address these issues, NMHCs will continue to be underutilized, and the full potential of the NMHC model will not be realized.

The success NMHCs had in getting inserted into the ACA and the IOM report is, however, a clear example of what advocates can do when they remain politically active and strategic about forming alliances. NNCC's policy team and other nursing organizations are working to keep the pressure on policy makers so that the reforms and recommendations called for in the ACA and the IOM report can be achieved. As mentioned earlier, some key initiatives currently being pursued include (a) the push to get the NMHC grant program reauthorized and funded and (b) the attempt to craft a new graduate nurse education demonstration project that places greater emphasis on providing nursing students with clinical placements in NMHCs. These two programs could potentially benefit NMHCs across the county, but to make them a reality, nurses, nursing students, and nurse advocates of every level need to engage in the political process.

REFERENCES

Congressional Budget Office. (2014). *Updated estimates of the effects of the insurance coverage provisions of the affordable care act, April 2014.* Retrieved from http://www.cbo.gov/sites/default/files/cbofiles/attachments/45231-ACA_Estimates.pdf

Fairman, J., & Okoye, S. (2011). Nursing for the future from the past: two reports from the institute of medicine. *Journal of Nursing Education, 50*(6), 305–311.

Hansen-Turton, T., Miller, M., & Grenier, P. (2009). *Nurse-managed wellness centers: Developing and maintaining your center.* New York, NY: Springer Publishing Company.

Hansen-Turton, T., Ware, J., Bond, L., Doria, N., & Cunningham, P. (2013). Are managed care organizations in the united states impeding the delivery of primary care by nurse practitioners? A 2012 update on managed care organization credentialing and reimbursement practices. *Population Health Management, 16*(5), 306–309.

Institute of Medicine (IOM). (2010). *The future of nursing: Leading change, advancing health.* Retrieved from http://www.aamn.org/docs/future-of-nursing.pdf

National Nursing Centers Consortium (NNCC). (2012). *Prevention and public health fund dollars and nurse-managed clinics.* Philadelphia, PA: NNCC Policy Education Center. Retrieved from http://www.nncc.us/site/images/pdf/policy/PreventionandPublicHealthFundDollarsandNMHC_2012.pdf

Patient Protection and Affordable Care Act, Pub. L. No. 111-148, § 5208, 612 Stat. 124 (2010a).

Patient Protection and Affordable Care Act, Pub. L. No. 111-148, § 5316, 995 Stat. 124 (2010b).

Patient Protection and Affordable Care Act, Pub. L. No. 111-148, § 5509, 674 Stat. 124 (2010c).

The White House. (n.d.). *The Obama administration's record on supporting the nursing workforce.* Retrieved from http://www.whitehouse.gov/sites/default/files/docs/nurses_report_0.pdf

Wood, D. (2013). Progress implementing the IOM's future of nursing recommendations. *Nurse Zone.* Retrieved from http://www.nursezone.com/Nursing-News-Events/more-news/Progress-Implementing-the-IOMs-Future-of-Nursing-Recommendations_41897.aspx

CHAPTER 17

Health Care Transformations and The Future of Nursing: Campaign for Action

Susan B. Hassmiller

It is an incredibly exciting time to be involved in health care. The health and health care fields are undergoing a much-needed transformation to promote wellness and serve more people better. Nurse-managed clinics, primary care medical homes, and other innovations offer promising solutions to some of the most pressing health challenges our country faces, including an aging and more diverse population with more chronic conditions, soaring costs, and a shortage of providers.

The Institute of Medicine's (IOM's) landmark report *The Future of Nursing: Leading Change, Advancing Health* offers important and timely recommendations to help our country meet these challenges by zeroing in on how strengthening the nursing profession could help to improve health for patients, families, and communities. As the largest segment of the health care workforce—and the ones who spend the most time with patients and their families—nurses are vital to reforming our health system to improve outcomes and support a culture of health. The report offers detailed recommendations on ways to strengthen the nursing field to improve health and health care for everyone in America.

The Robert Wood Johnson Foundation (RWJF), the nation's largest health care philanthropy, and AARP, the nation's largest consumer organization, realized immediately that the IOM recommendations, if implemented, could help to address many of the issues that plague our nation as well as to expand access to care, improve quality, and help contain health care costs for millions of Americans. In 2011, shortly after the report's release, RWJF and AARP launched The Future of Nursing: Campaign for Action to implement these recommendations. Nurse leaders in all 50 states and the District of Columbia partnered with other health professionals, hospitals and health systems, community groups, business leaders, philanthropy, policy makers, and other health care leaders to improve health through nursing. The campaign's vision is to ensure that everyone in America can live a healthier life, supported by a system in which nurses are essential partners in providing care and promoting health. These state-based action coalitions are working to promote nursing leadership, remove barriers to practice, strengthen nursing education, foster interprofessional collaboration, and improve workforce diversity.

The Future of Nursing Scholars program is another major initiative that grew out of the IOM report and is funded by RWJF and other stakeholders. In 2013, the foundation pledged $20 million and invited other stakeholders to join them to increase the number of nurses with PhDs. This program is in direct response to the IOM recommendation to double the number of nurses with doctorate degrees. The program aims, in particular, to replenish an aging nurse faculty pool and increase the cadre of nurse scientists, innovators, and policy makers to improve patient care. Based at the University of Pennsylvania, the program selected its inaugural cohort of schools (who chose their scholars) in 2014.

Many of the IOM recommendations will take years to implement, but the campaign has begun to record successes. Since it began, seven states have removed barriers to advanced practice registered nurse practice and care. In 2013, 15 states introduced legislation to ensure that these nurses could practice to the full extent of their education and training. Several editorial boards, including *The New York Times* and *Bloomberg*, have called for the removal of these barriers, and public opinion is shifting in favor of removing barriers to practice. Seventeen states are streamlining the education process to make it easier for nurses to advance from an associate's degree to a bachelor's degree in nursing, and there was a 27% increase in Doctor of Nursing Practice enrollments and a 4% increase in PhD nursing enrollments from 2011 to 2012. In addition, nine state action coalitions have filled 41 state leadership positions with nurses. Several major institutions are working on interprofessional collaboration programs, and progress is being made on the workforce data front and in making the nursing workforce more diverse.

If you are not already involved, join the Campaign for Action and work to improve care in your community and state. Go to www.campaignforaction. org to sign up. Let us work together to help ensure that all people get the care they need, when they need it.

Nurse-Managed Health Clinic Start-Up Checklist

Checklist	Questions to Think About	Advice From Experts
Getting 501(c)(3) status	Will the health center be an independent 501(c)(3) or will it operate under the umbrella of another nonprofit entity?	• Having its own 501(c)(3) status allows a center greater financial freedom and the opportunity to obtain FQHC status. Information on the process of filing for 501(c)(3) status can be found at the IRS website www.irs.gov/ charities/ index.html
Create a governing or advisory board	What kind of skills do you need to start out? Who do you know who has these skills? What key community figures might be able to help?	• A board should comprise a group of dedicated people to share tasks and problem solve. Health center users are required to comprise a minimum of 51% of an FQHC's board. In addition to health center users, board members may be health center partners or experts in fund-raising, legal issues, and quality of care. • Find others in the community doing similar work and utilize them as resources. Job descriptions should reflect the mission.
Mission statement	What is the primary goal of the health center? What is the guiding principle behind starting the health center?	• The mission helps guide decision making and articulate the health center's vision to funders, staff, and patients. • Keep it short and clear.

(continued)

(continued)

Checklist	Questions to Think About	Advice From Experts
Needs assessment	Who in the community will be the target population? What is the community population profile? What is the status of the existing health care delivery system? What will be the health center's range of services?	• Start with existing data—such as U.S. Census, local health department, local United Way, or local hospital data—to gain a better understanding of the community's needs.
Rules and regulations	What are the state, city, and local laws that pertain?	• Being well informed about rules and regulations will help prevent malpractice and other legal problems.
Resource assessment	What services are other agencies in the area providing? Are there any gaps in the service? What are the eligibility requirements for Medicare and Medicaid?	• This will help determine the types of services the health center should offer and will help identify potential partnerships and referral sources.
Finance	How much money is needed to start the health center? How and where will the center seek donations and grants? How will the billing system work?	• This will guide the services that the center will provide and will help identify gaps.
Insurance	What types of insurance will the center need? What types of liability coverage will the practitioners need?	• There are two types of liability coverage: professional liability insurance for the provider and comprehensive general liability for the facility. • Under the Federally Supported Health Centers Assistance Act, health centers funded under Section 330 of the Public Health Service Act are eligible for medical malpractice insurance at no cost to the grantee (Federal Tort Claim Act). • Other health centers will need to purchase private professional liability insurance. Requirements vary from state to state; see www.hpso.com

(continued)

Checklist	Questions to Think About	Advice From Experts
Space and site selection	Is the location in a medically underserved area, a health professional shortage area, or an area with a special medically underserved population? Where should the center be located to be most accessible to the target population? How many rooms and offices are needed? Is a conference room necessary?	• It is key to locate services in an area of need and to avoid duplicating existing services. Duplication will handicap the center's ability to receive grants and FQHC status. • Take into consideration the number of clients to be served, how much space is needed for exam or meeting rooms and offices, and access by public transportation. • Generally, one primary care clinician needs a minimum of two exam rooms to maximize productivity.
Staffing	How many practitioners and support staff does the health center need to operate? Does the center need volunteers, and how will they be recruited? What credentials are required?	• Generally, a ratio of two to three support staff (MA, RN, or LPN, front desk) per full-time clinician will allow for 16–22 patient visits.
Business operations	What hours of operation are needed? What type of call system will be set up to ensure that patients have 24-hour access to providers where necessary?	• What are state regulations regarding payers contracting with independent NPs? • Expectations for an FQHC are a minimum of 20 hours per week, 52 weeks a year. • Twenty-four-hour telephone coverage is required for primary care.
Licenses and Approvals	Is all of the necessary paperwork completed to comply with relevant state and federal requirements? What equipment is needed? Is a laboratory needed?	• The state and federal governments must approve all practices, even those with small labs. • Clinical Laboratory Improvement Amendments (CLIA) certification is required for all labs. A lab limited to performing "waived" tests is subject to less regulation. Waived tests include, but are not limited to, Hct or Hgb, urine dipstick, urine pregnancy test, fingerstick blood sugars and hemoccult, and vaginal wet smears. Waived tests may vary; regulations may change as new reliable tests become available. (www.cms.hhs.gov/clia)

(continued)

(continued)

Checklist	Questions to Think About	Advice From Experts
Credentialing, quality improvement/ quality assurance	What is the credentialing process in the particular service area? How will the center measure the quality of care that the patients receive?	• Advanced practice nurses must be properly certified. This is essential for credentialing by MCOs and it helps prevent successful malpractice suits. All primary care, behavioral health, and specialty providers must be credentialed. Searching the National Practitioner Data Bank (www.npdb.hrsa.gov) is advisable. • A system must be in place to maintain patient quality of care and health center management. A QI committee should be established. • The NNCC Quality Management Document is a helpful resource and is available on the NNCC website.

Sample Nurse-Managed Health Clinic Bylaws

_____Health Center, Incorporated
Bylaws

ARTICLE I

Principal Office

The principal office of the Corporation shall be at _____,
_____ or such other location within the State of _____
as the Board of Directors may determine from time to time.

ARTICLE 2

Purposes

The purposes of the Corporation are to own, operate, and maintain a health
center for the study, diagnosis, and treatment of human ailments and injuries; to promote medical, surgical, and scientific research and learning; and
such other purposes as may be pursued in accordance with the Certificate
of Incorporation, as in effect from time to time. These purposes for which
the Corporation organized are exclusively charitable, scientific, literary, and
educational within the meaning of Section 501(c)(3) of the Internal Revenue
Code of 1986 or the corresponding provision of any future United States
Internal Revenue Service law.

Notwithstanding any other provision of these articles, this organization shall not carry on any activities not permitted to be carried on by an organization exempt from federal income tax under Section 501(c)(3) of the Internal Revenue Code of 1986 or the corresponding provision of any future United States Internal Revenue Service law.

ARTICLE 3

Directors

1. *Powers.* The activities, property, and affairs of the Corporation shall be managed by the Board of Directors. It may adopt such rules and regulations as may be required by regulatory authorities.
2. *Elections of Directors.* The initial Board of Directors shall be elected by the incorporator(s). Thereafter, directorships vacant or to be vacant at an Annual Meeting shall be filled by the election of the required number of directors from the candidates nominated in accordance with Paragraph 5 of this Article. Upon demand of any two directors in person, elections shall be conducted by written ballot.
3. *Number and Term of Office.* The Board of Directors shall consist of 11 persons. The number of directorships shall be determined at each Annual Meeting of the Board and from time to time by the Board of Directors. The terms of the directors shall be so fixed that the terms of one third of such directors shall expire at each Annual Meeting of the Corporation. Approximately one third of the directors shall be elected each year for a three-year term. No director may serve more than two consecutive terms or six consecutive years.
4. *Composition of the Board.* At least 51% of the directors must be individuals who utilize the services of the health center as their medical or dental home and be known as users of the Corporation. The remaining members, known as non-users of the Board, shall complement the user members of the Board in terms of technical expertise in areas such as finance, health care delivery, business, law, education, community relations, religion, and investments. Such technical expertise is appropriate to provide oversight to center operations and activities. No more than one half of the non-user members of the Board may earn more than 10% of their income from the health field.
5. *Nomination and Election of Directors.* Not less than sixty (60) days prior to each Annual Meeting, the Board of Directors shall elect a Nominations Committee of three (3) directors, who shall determine the number of

directorships for the following year. The Nominations Committee, acting by unanimous vote, shall nominate a number of nominees for director equal to the number of directorships that are vacant or will become vacant at the Annual Meeting. In making such nominations, the Nominations Committee shall take into account the requirements concerning the composition of the Board set forth in Paragraph 4 of this Article.

6. Not less than thirty (30) days before each Annual Meeting, the Nominations Committee shall submit to the Secretary its nominations for directors, and the Secretary shall immediately inform the Board of Directors of these nominations. Not less than fourteen (14) days before the Annual Meeting, any five (5) directors, including at least one consumer/user member, may submit to the Secretary the names of one or more additional nominees ("Alternative Nominees") for director, each of whom shall be designated by them as being alternatives to one of the Nominations Committee Nominees. At the Annual Meeting, the voting procedure followed shall be such that a separate vote is taken for each directorship to be filled, each Nominations Committee Nominee being matched with his/her respective Alternative Nominee(s). Each directorship shall be filled by majority vote of the directors voting (a quorum must be present), except that no nominee may be elected if the effect of such election would be to cause the composition of the Board to be in violation of the requirements contained in Paragraph 4 of this Article.

7. *Expiration of Terms.* Notwithstanding any other provision contained in these Bylaws, the term of office of any director shall not expire until his successor has been duly elected and has agreed to serve.

8. *Vacancies.* When any directorship becomes vacant during the period between Annual Meetings of the Corporation, the directors may elect a new director to fill such vacancy until the next Annual Meeting. At such Annual Meeting, such directorship shall be filled as provided in Paragraphs 4 and 5 of this Article and for such term as may be appropriate.

9. Nominations to fill such vacancies shall be made by the Nominations Committee, with additional nominations being permitted from the floor.

10. *Director Compensation.* No member of the Board of Directors shall be compensated for his or her service on the Board, although he or she may be reimbursed for reasonable and necessary expenses incurred for the benefit of the Corporation. Reimbursement shall require the submission of expense vouchers and receipts per corporate travel policies.

11. *Nepotism.* No employee or relative of an employee by blood or marriage may serve as a member of the Board of Directors. Relative is defined as mother, father, sister, brother, aunt, uncle, grandmother, grandfather, and first cousin.

ARTICLE 4

Meetings

1. *Regular Meetings.* The Board of Directors shall hold regular monthly meetings pursuant to a resolution of the Board establishing the meeting schedule. If the Board fails to establish such a schedule providing otherwise, it shall hold regular monthly meetings on the fourth _____ of each month. Said meetings shall be held pursuant to written notice given to each director not less than five (5) days before the time set for the meeting, such written notification to include the agenda.

2. *Special Meetings.* Special meetings may be called by the President or by any three directors contacting the President. Special meetings shall be held within or outside of the State of _____.

   a. *Telephonic Communication.* Members of the Board of Directors may participate in any meeting of the Board by means of conference telephone or similar communications equipment that enables all participants in the meeting to hear each other at the same time. Such participation shall constitute presence in person at the meeting.

3. *Quorum and Voting.* A majority of the directors seated shall constitute a quorum for the transaction of business at any directors' meeting, whether annual, regular, or special. If a quorum is present, the act of a majority of directors voting shall be an act of the Board of Directors, except as otherwise expressly provided in these bylaws.

   a. *Notice.* Notice shall be given in writing to each director of each annual, regular, or special meeting of the directors. Such notice shall be delivered by hand, by mail, or by facsimile at least five (5) days before an annual or regular meeting and at least one (1) day before a special meeting. The notice shall state the date, time, place, and purpose of the meeting.

   b. *Waiver of Notice.* A written waiver signed by a director, or attendance by a director at any annual, regular, or special meeting, shall be deemed equivalent to appropriate notice and shall be deemed consent to the holding of the meeting.

c. *Attendance.* Any director who fails to be present at three regular meetings of the Board in succession or five (5) for the year, regardless of the reason for the absence, may be removed as a director by the affirmative vote of a majority of the other members of the Board. Any director may also be removed for cause by two-thirds (2/3) vote of the members entitled to vote.

d. *Conflicts of Interest.* The Corporation shall avoid the active participation of any director in a manner that poses a conflict of interest with respect to that director. A conflict of interest shall be considered to arise when any matter under consideration by the Board of Directors involves the potential for a significant or material benefit; or a compensation arrangement exists between a director or any member of his or her immediate family and any business, financial, or professional organization of which the director or any member of his or her immediate family is an officer, director, member, owner, or employee. Whenever any matter comes before the Board of Directors which any director recognizes may give rise to a conflict of interest, the Board of Directors shall not approve any action or transaction bearing upon the conflict unless the following procedures are observed:

1) The affected director or other director(s) shall make known the conflict, and after answering any questions posed by the other directors, the affected director shall withdraw from the meeting for as long as the matter remains under consideration. Should the matter be brought to a vote of the directors, the affected director shall neither be present nor cast a vote.

2) If the withdrawal of the affected director results in the absence of a quorum, no action shall be taken on the matter until a quorum of disinterested directors is present.

The Board of Directors shall not go forward with a transaction or arrangement in which an affected director acknowledges that a conflict of interest exists, or other directors determine that a conflict of interest exists.

ARTICLE 5

Officers

1. *Officers.* The officers of the Corporation shall be a President, a Vice-President, a Treasurer, a Secretary, and Executive Director and such other officers as the Board of Directors may from time to time elect. The duties of

the officers of the Corporation shall be as provided in this Article, except as modified from time to time by the Board.

2. *Nomination and Election.* The Nominations Committee shall present nominations for the offices of President, Vice President, Secretary, and Treasurer at each Annual Meeting and at other times when vacancies occur in the offices. Additional nominations may be made from the floor. The President, Vice-President, Secretary, and Treasurer shall be members of the Board and shall be elected to serve for a term of one year and until their successors are duly elected and have agreed to serve.

3. *President.* The President shall preside at meetings of the Board, shall have general responsibility for dealing with questions of policy related to the Corporation's affairs and shall be responsible for calling meetings of the Board and for assuring adequate communication between the operating staff of the Corporation and the Board on matters of policy.

4. *Vice-President.* The Vice-President shall perform such duties as may from time to time be assigned to him/her by the Board of Directors or designated to him/her by the President. In case of the death, disability, or absence of the President, he/she shall fulfill all the duties and be vested with all powers and responsibilities of the President.

5. *Secretary.* The Secretary shall keep a book of minutes of all meetings of the Board, shall issue all notices required by Law or requested from time-to-time by the Board of Directors or by the President, and shall perform such other duties as are incident to the office of Secretary. He/she shall have custody of the seal of this Corporation and all books, records, and papers of this Corporation, except such as shall be in the charge of the Treasurer, Clinical Director, or of some other person authorized to have custody and possession thereof by a resolution of the Board of Directors.

6. *Treasurer.* The Treasurer serves as the principal financial advisor to the Board of Directors in planning, directing and appraising the effectiveness of _____ Health Center's fiscal operations. The Treasurer shall ensure full and accurate accountability and control of the receipts and disbursements of _____ Health Center's assets. The Treasurer shall perform such other duties as may be assigned by the Board of Directors or as are incidental to the office.

7. *Executive Director.* The Executive Director shall be appointed or dismissed by the Board of Directors, shall be an ex-officio member of the Board of Directors, and as the Chief Executive Officer of the Corporation, shall direct all operations of the Corporation; shall supervise all personnel; and shall have control and management of its business and affairs, all subject

to the direction of the Board of Directors. The Board shall evaluate the performance of the Executive Director annually, against a set of written, agreed-upon goals and objectives.

8. *Appointment of Staff.* The medical and dental staff of the Corporation shall be appointed at each Annual Meeting by vote of the Board.

ARTICLE 6

Committees

1. *Committees.* Standing committees of the Corporation shall include an Executive Committee, a Nominations Committee, a Finance Committee, an Operations Committee, a Bylaws Committee, and a Continuous Quality Improvement Committee. The President, subject to the approval of the Board of Directors, shall appoint members to committees for a term of one year and until their successors have been elected and have agreed to serve. At each Annual Meeting, the Board of Directors may appoint other special committees as circumstances may require.

2. *Service on Committee.* The President, subject to the approval of the Board of Directors, shall appoint the chairperson and members of all committees, except as otherwise provided by these Bylaws. Every standing committee and special committee shall include at least one Board member. The terms of office of committee chairpersons and members shall be for one year or until the end of the Annual Meeting following their appointment. No person shall serve more than three successive years as committee chairperson, but there shall be no limitation on the length of time individuals may serve as members of a committee. The President and the Executive Director shall be ex-officio members of all committees except as otherwise provided in these Bylaws.

3. *The Executive Committee.* The Board of Directors shall elect an Executive Committee. The members thereof shall be the President, who shall serve as chairman of the committee; the Vice-President; Secretary; Treasurer; and one additional director, who must be a consumer member director. Said one additional member shall be elected to the Executive Committee at each Annual Meeting following the election of directors and shall serve for a meeting; the Nominations Committee shall present nominations for the positions on the Executive Committee to be filled. The Executive Committee shall have power and authority to take actions on behalf of the Board of Directors for emergencies that occur between meetings of the Board. It is intended that the Executive Committee not be utilized

to conduct the business of the Board. All actions taken by the Executive Committee shall be reported at the next meeting of the Board and shall be binding on the Board only when approved by formal vote of the Board.

4. *Nominations Committee.* The membership of the Nominations Committee shall consist of three (3) Board members appointed by the President. The Nominations Committee shall present nominations for vacancies on the Board and for the offices of President, Vice-President, Secretary, and Treasurer at each Annual Meeting and at other times when vacancies occur in the offices. The Nominations Committee will assure that new Board members receive an orientation to the Health Center and to the role and responsibilities of membership on the Board of Directors.

5. *Finance Committee.*
   a. Membership—The membership of the Finance Committee shall consist of the Treasurer and three (3) Board members appointed by the President of the Board of Directors.
   b. Functions—The Finance Committee shall be responsible to the Board of Directors for the fiscal affairs of the Corporation. Such responsibilities include:
      1) Review, monitor, and approve program budget and recommend changes;
      2) Review and recommend policies regarding financial management activities;
      3) Review and approve all purchases over $5,000;
      4) Review and report to the Board on all internal and external audits;
      5) Report to the Board of Directors on _____ Health Center's financial activities; and
      6) Perform other functions as requested of the committees by the President of the Board of Directors.
   c. Meetings—The Finance Committee shall meet at least once each month for the purpose of reviewing monthly financial statements.
   d. Quorum—Three (3) members of the Finance Committee shall constitute a quorum.

6. *Operations Committee.* The Operations Committee shall have oversight responsibilities for the development of personnel policies, job qualifications, rates of pay, vacation, and employee benefits, as well as the Strategic Plan and decisions about grant applications and new services. The Operations Committee shall make recommendations concerning the general layout for the physical plant in accordance with the functional needs of the Corporation and shall have general supervision of the upkeep and maintenance of the Corporation's buildings and grounds. This committee

shall have the responsibility for reviewing contracts entered into by the Corporation. Members of the committee shall prepare for negotiations by becoming familiar with existing contracts at _____ Health Center and current contracts at similar facilities, and developing a knowledge of proper labor management principles and practices.

7. *Bylaws Committee.* The Bylaws Committee shall make recommendations for changes and revisions to the Bylaws to the Board of Directors and shall meet with a frequency dictated by need or otherwise determined by the Board of Directors.

8. *Continuous Quality Improvement Committee.* The Continuous Quality Improvement (CQI) Committee shall develop a system designed to maintain the quality of health care rendered, including a periodic audit of patient records conducted with sufficient frequency to adequately monitor the continuing quality of such care. The CQI Committee will review, approve, and revise as necessary a continuous quality improvement and quality management program commensurate with AMA, ADA, OSHA, and all local, state, and federal regulations. The CQI Committee will also periodically conduct a review of the Board's own performance. The CQI Committee shall meet at least quarterly, or four (4) times per year.

ARTICLE 7

Dissolution

Upon the dissolution of the Corporation, assets shall be distributed for one or more exempt purposes within the meaning of Section 501(c)(3) of the Internal Revenue Code of 1986, or corresponding section of any future federal tax code, or shall be distributed to the federal government, or to a state or local government, for a public purpose. Any such assets not so disposed of shall be disposed of by the Court of Common Pleas of the county in which the principal office of the Corporation is then located, exclusively for such purposes or to such organization or organizations, as said Court shall determine, which are organized and operated exclusively for such purposes.

ARTICLE 8

Amendments

The directors may, by a two-thirds vote of those present in person at any duly called meeting at which a quorum is represented, alter, amend, or repeal these Bylaws or any portion thereof except that Paragraphs 4 and 5 of Article

3 may be altered, amended, or repealed only by the affirmative vote of four-fifths of the directors present.

Written notice as to the substance and effect of any proposed amendment to the Bylaws shall be given or mailed to each director not less than thirty (30) days prior to the meeting of the Board at which such proposed amendment is submitted to a vote.

ADOPTED BY THE BOARD OF DIRECTORS ON _____.

_____

President Date

Board of Directors

THE NATIONAL NURSING CENTERS CONSORTIUM MANAGED CARE CONTRACTING TOOLKIT

Tine Hansen-Turton

INSTRUCTIONS

As a result of work done under a Samuel Fels Foundation grant, the National Nursing Centers Consortium (NNCC) has found that, despite favorable legal authority, many health insurance companies are not contracting with nurse practitioners (NPs) as primary care providers (PCPs) individually or as specialists. Each company follows its own business decisions, and therefore carriers in the same state can have different policies. We are trying to assess which companies are contracting with NPs; if they are not, we are trying to determine what and where the stumbling blocks are. This health insurance company contracting toolkit is intended to walk you through the contracting process in a user-friendly way. Our goal is to support your being credentialed and reimbursed by health insurers for your services, making NPs a financially sustainable part of the safety net. We need you to help us build a record of which insurance companies, in what markets, continue to resist contracting with NPs in nurse-managed health clinics. NNCC will then move forward with contacting those insurance companies to educate and try, in a focused way, to change their NP contracting policies. Please pursue PCP status with your local insurance companies *now*.

STEP 1—SECTION A: STATE-BY-STATE POLICY GUIDE

Locate your state and look to see which level of physician involvement is required for your state.

STEP 2—SECTION B: EXPLANATION OF EACH LEVEL OF PHYSICIAN INVOLVEMENT

A. Introduction

The purpose of this memorandum is to provide examples of how various states regulate physician involvement in NP practices. There are basically four ways states have chosen to regulate the physician collaboration aspect of NP practice: (a) Some states allow NPs to practice independent of any physician oversight; (b) some states require an NP to enter into a collaborative agreement with a physician before he or she can practice; (c) some states require the physician to delegate authority to the NP before the NP can practice; and (d) some states require the physician to provide supervision before the NP can practice. This memorandum examines how the states have set up these different practice models by looking at the regulatory scheme used by one state from each of the four categories. A fifth category is included to highlight regulations that exist in some states that use some combination of the above to regulate physician involvement. The example given here is Pennsylvania, which has enacted regulations that, on their face, call for physician supervision, but in practice, follow a model more based on NP–physician collaboration.

B. Independent Practice

An example of a state that permits independent practice is New Hampshire. The regulations governing the advanced registered nurse practitioner (ARNP) scope of practice state:

(a) "The ARNP shall be competent as set forth below to practice independently in a variety of settings.
(b) The ARNP shall have the ability to
  (1) Elicit and record physical and mental health status, psychosocial history, including review of bodily systems;
  (2) Perform physical examination;
  (3) Initiate appropriate diagnostic tests to screen or evaluate the care recipient's current health status;

(4) Assess findings of history, review of systems, physical examination and diagnostic tests, and formulate a diagnosis prior to implementing a treatment regimen;

(5) Identify health problems and learning needs of the care recipient;

(6) Plan, teach, promote and manage physical and mental health care in a continuous program;

(7) Implement and manage treatment regimens and administer, prescribe, dispense and procure pharmacological agents;

(8) Arrange appropriate referrals;

(9) Initiate appropriate emergency treatment in life-threatening or unusual situations in order to stabilize the care recipient; and

(10) Provide other functions common to the nurse practitioner, certified nurse midwife, certified registered nurse anesthetist or psychiatric/mental-health specialist role for which the ARNP is educationally and experientially prepared" (N.H. CODE ADMIN. R. ANN. [NUR] 300.304.05).

In addition, the statute governing ARNP prescriptive authority in New Hampshire states:

"An ARNP shall have plenary authority to possess, compound, prescribe, administer, and dispense and distribute to clients controlled and non-controlled drugs in accordance with the formulary established by the joint health council and within the scope of the ARNP's practice as defined by this chapter. Such authority may be denied, suspended, or revoked by the board after notice and the opportunity for hearing, upon proof that the authority has been abused" (N.H. REV. STAT. ANN. § 326-B:11).

As with most other states in which NPs practice independently, New Hampshire does not have any formal NP–physician collaboration requirement in its statutes or regulations. The law further highlights the autonomous nature of NP practice by using terms like "practice independently" and "plenary authority" when describing an NP's scope of practice and ability to prescribe medication.

C. Collaboration

The majority of states mandate that an NP enter into a collaborative agreement with a licensed physician before beginning practice at an independent site. These agreements are typically developed with the input of both the NP and the physician. They usually cover a few basic areas of practice such

as the functions the NP can perform, referral and consultation procedures, prescriptive authority, and quality assurance measures. A good example of a state that follows a collaboration model is Maryland, which mandates that
"Before a nurse practitioner may practice he shall:...

(2) Enter into a written agreement with a physician whereby the physician on a regularly-scheduled basis shall:
   (a) Accept referrals,
   (b) Establish and review drug and other medical guidelines with the nurse practitioner,
   (c) Participate with the nurse practitioner in periodically reviewing and discussing medical diagnoses and the therapeutic or corrective measures employed in the practice setting,
   (d) Jointly sign records if needed to document accountability of both the physician and nurse practitioner,
   (e) Be available for consultation in person, by telephone, or by some other form of telecommunication, and
   (f) Designate an alternate physician if the physician identified in the written agreement temporarily becomes unavailable" (Code Md. Regs. tit. 10, § 10.27.07.02[2][b], LEXIS, current through June 9, 2006).

The regulations mentioned specifically govern the establishment of a collaborative practice, but Maryland law also references the fact that an NP must enter into a written collaboration agreement with a physician in both the regulation governing NP scope of practice and the regulation governing NP prescriptive authority. Therefore, the wording of the collaboration agreement will have an impact on the degree of independence the NP may exercise.

On their faces, the regulations governing the establishment of collaborative agreements may appear to give the collaborating physician a great deal of control over an NP practice. However, NPs practicing in states that follow collaborative models do experience a considerable measure of professional autonomy. For example, in Maryland, physicians must be available to accept referrals and consultations from the NP, but this stipulation does not require the physician to be physically present at the NP's practice site. The NP is able to fulfill the consultation requirement through any form of telecommunication.

D. Delegation

Some states require an NP to obtain delegated authority from a physician before beginning practice at an independent site. In practice, a delegation model functions much the same as a collaboration model. The delegated authority is most often centered around prescriptive authority, as is the case with the Michigan regulation cited in the following text. Michigan law specifically states that

(1) "A physician may delegate the prescription of controlled substances listed in schedules 3 to 5 to a registered nurse who holds specialty certification under section 17210 of the code, with the exception of a nurse anesthetist, if the delegating physician establishes a written authorization that contains all of the following information:
   (a) The name, license number, and signature of the delegating physician.
   (b) The name, license number, and signature of the nurse practitioner or nurse midwife.
   (c) The limitations or exceptions to the delegation.
   (d) The effective date of the delegation.
(2) A delegating physician shall review and update a written authorization on an annual basis from the original date or the date of amendment, if amended. A delegating physician shall note the review date on the written authorization.
(3) A delegating physician shall maintain a written authorization in each separate location of the physician's office where the delegation occurs.
(4) A delegating physician shall ensure that an amendment to the written authorization is in compliance with subrule (1) (a) to (d) of this rule.
(5) A delegating physician may delegate the prescription of schedule 2 controlled substances only if all of the following conditions are met:
   (a) The delegating physician and nurse practitioner or nurse midwife are practicing within a health facility as defined in section 20106(d), (g), or (i) of the code; specifically, freestanding surgical outpatient facilities, hospitals, and hospices.
   (b) The patient is located within the facility described in subdivision (a) of this subrule.
   (c) The delegation is in compliance with this rule.
(6) A delegating physician may not delegate the prescription of schedule 2 controlled substances issued for the discharge of a patient for a quantity for more than a 7-day period.
(7) A delegating physician shall not delegate the prescription of a drug or device individually, in combination, or in succession for a woman known to be pregnant with the intention of causing either a miscarriage or fetal death" (Mich. Admin. Code. r. 338.2305, LEXIS, current through June 23, 2006).

In Michigan, the requirements for the delegation agreement are much the same as the requirements that might be found in a typical collaboration agreement. Michigan law states that the delegation agreement should be in writing, especially if the NP is going to prescribe Schedule 3, 4, or 5 controlled substances. Any written agreement, or amendment thereto, must have the name and license number of the physician and NP and the effective date of the writing, and any limitations or exceptions to the delegations and the agreement must be reviewed and updated annually.

In some cases, a delegation practice model may give the physician more control over an NP practice and over what is included in the delegation agreement because the physician is free to delegate at his or her discretion. For example, Michigan requires prescriptions written by NPs to bear the name of the delegating physician (Mich. Comp. Laws r333.17048[5], LEXIS, current through June 12, 2006). However, the discretion granted the physician by the delegation practice model does not substantially limit the amount of autonomy enjoyed by NPs in delegation states.

Michigan law still does not require the delegating physician to be present at the practice site. Neither are delegating physicians required to provide direct on-site supervision in California, another delegation state. The consultation requirement can be fulfilled through telecommunication contact.

E. Supervision

Some states characterize the level of physician involvement in NP practices as amounting to physician supervision. For example, Tennessee requires that a licensed physician supervise the practice of an NP. The law states:

"It is the intent of these rules to maximize the collaborative practice of certified nurse practitioners and supervising physicians in a manner consistent with quality health care delivery.

(1) A supervising physician, certified nurse practitioner or a substitute supervising physician must possess a current, unencumbered license to practice in the state of Tennessee.

(2) Supervision does not require the continuous and constant presence of the supervising physician; however, the supervising physician must be available for consultation at all times or shall make arrangements for a substitute physician to be available.

(3) A supervising physician and/or substitute supervising physician shall have experience and/or expertise in the same area of medicine as the certified nurse practitioner.

(4) Nurse Practitioners who hold a temporary certificate of fitness shall be supervised pursuant to T.C.A. § 63-7-123 and Board of Nursing rule 1000-4-.04. Such supervision requires the physical presence of either the supervising physician or certified nurse practitioner.

(5) Protocols are required and:

    (a) Shall be jointly developed and approved by the supervising physician and nurse practitioner;

    (b) Shall outline and cover the applicable standard of care;

    (c) Shall be reviewed and updated biennially;

    (d) Shall be maintained at the practice site;

    (e) Shall account for all protocol drugs by appropriate formulary;

    (f) Shall be specific to the population seen;

    (g) Shall be dated and signed; and

    (h) Copies of protocols and formularies shall be maintained at the practice site and shall be made available upon request for inspection by the respective boards.

(6) The supervising physician shall be responsible for ensuring compliance with the applicable standard of care under (5).

Additionally, the supervising physician shall develop clinical guidelines in collaboration with the certified nurse practitioner to include a method for documenting consultation and referral.

(7) Once every ten (10) business days the supervising physician shall make a personal review of the historical, physical and therapeutic data and shall so certify by signature on any patient within thirty (30) days:

    (a) When medically indicated;

    (b) When requested by the patient;

    (c) When prescriptions written by the certified nurse practitioner fall outside the protocols;

    (d) When prescriptions are written by a nurse practitioner who possesses a temporary certificate of fitness; and

    (e) When a controlled drug has been prescribed.

(8) In any event, a supervising physician shall personally review at least twenty percent (20%) of charts monitored or written by the certified nurse practitioner every thirty (30) days.

(9) The supervising physician shall be required to visit any remote site at least once every thirty (30) days.

(10) Any prescription written and signed or drug issued by a nurse practitioner under the supervision and control of a supervising physician shall be deemed to be that of the nurse practitioner.

(11) The supervising physician shall make provision for preprinted prescription pads bearing the name, address and telephone number of the supervising physician and that of the nurse practitioner. The nurse practitioner shall sign his or her own name on each prescription so written. Where the preprinted prescription pad contains the names of more than one (1) physician, the nurse practitioner shall indicate on the prescription which of those physicians is the nurse practitioner's primary supervising physician by placing a checkmark beside or a circle around the name of that physician.

(12) Eligible certified nurse practitioners shall use numbers assigned to them by the DEA when prescribing controlled substances" (Tenn. Comp. R. & Regs.0880-6-.02, LEXIS, current through May 2006).

Again, the use of the term "supervision" does not call for any greater level of physician involvement than would exist under a typical collaboration or delegation agreement. In Tennessee, the agreement entered into by a physician and an NP, which is called a protocol, essentially covers the same areas as a delegation agreement in Michigan (cited in the preceding text).

With regard to prescriptive authority, the Tennessee statute provides:

"A nurse who has been issued a certificate of fitness as a nurse practitioner pursuant to [Tenn. Code Ann.] § 63-7-207 and this section shall file a notice with the board, containing the name of the nurse practitioner, the name of the licensed physician having supervision, control and responsibility for prescriptive services rendered by the nurse practitioner, and a copy of the formulary describing the categories of legend drugs to be prescribed and/or issued by the nurse practitioner. The nurse practitioner shall be responsible for updating this information.

(2) The nurse practitioner who holds a certificate of fitness shall be authorized to prescribe and/or issue controlled substances listed in Schedules II, III, IV and V of title 39, chapter 17, part 4, upon joint adoption of physician supervisory rules concerning controlled substances pursuant to subsection (d).

(3) (A) Any prescription written and signed or drug issued by a nurse practitioner under the supervision and control of a supervising physician shall be deemed to be that of the nurse practitioner. Every prescription issued by a nurse practitioner pursuant to this section shall be entered in the medical records of the patient and shall be written on a preprinted prescription pad bearing the name, address, and telephone number of the supervising physician and of the nurse practitioner, and

the nurse practitioner shall sign each prescription so written. Where the preprinted prescription pad contains the names of more than one (1) physician, the nurse practitioner shall indicate on the prescription which of those physicians is the nurse practitioner's primary supervising physician by placing a checkmark beside or a circle around the name of that physician" (Tenn. Code Ann. § 63-7-123[b], LEXIS, current through 2005 Sess.).

Finally, with regard to Tennessee, there has been some confusion as to whether NPs are allowed to diagnose. The confusion primarily comes from the way professional nursing is defined in the state's nurse practice act. The act currently defines professional nursing in a way that excludes professional nurses from performing acts of medical diagnosis and developing medical plans of care. Since NPs are professional nurses, this definition would seem to prohibit NPs from diagnosing, but this statute only applies to registered nurses, not advanced practice nurses (APNs) (Tenn. Code Ann. § 63-7-103[b], LEXIS current through 2005 Sess.).

The full text of the statute says, "The practice of professional nursing does not include acts of medical diagnosis or the development of a medical plan of care and therapeutics for a patient, except to the extent such acts may be authorized by §§ 63-1-132, 63-7-123 and 63-7-207." Sections 63-1-132, 63-7-123, and 63-7-207 of the Tennessee code specifically deal with NPs who prescribe medications. Given that the legislature went out of its way to exclude NPs from the requirements of 63-7-103(b), it would stand to reason that the statute only applies to registered nurses who have not gone on to obtain advanced practice certification. This conclusion is supported by the State Board of Nursing regulation 1000-4-.09, which requires APNs (with authority to prescribe) to make a diagnosis based on examinations and requires that all diagnostic and laboratory tests be consistent with good care (Tenn. Comp. R. & Regs. 1000-4-.09, 2006).

Furthermore, Tennessee law states:

"(a) 'Advanced practice nurse' means a registered nurse with a master's degree or higher in a nursing specialty and national specialty certification as a nurse practitioner, nurse anesthetist, nurse midwife, or clinical nurse specialist" (Tenn. Code Ann. § 63-7-126). By requiring nurse practitioners to obtain national certification, Tennessee is requiring them to be proficient in certain core competencies. One of these is the ability to diagnose. For example, the scope and standards of the American Academy of Nurse Practitioners includes the core competency of diagnosis as a component of its

NP certification. When taken in conjunction with the Board of Nurses regulation 1000-4-.09, the certification requirement shows that Tennessee law both implicitly and explicitly allows NPs to diagnose.

F. Pennsylvania: Supervision but Collaboration

The final category examined in this memorandum is states that use a combination of the previous language in their physician involvement statutes. Pennsylvania is one of these states; in its definition of NP, Pennsylvania regulations state that an NP "while functioning in the expanded role as a professional nurse, performs acts of medical diagnosis or prescription of medical therapeutic or corrective measures in collaboration with and under the direction of a physician licensed to practice medicine in this Commonwealth" (Pa. Code. tit. 49, § 21.251, LEXIS, current through Apr. 15, 2006). The term "direction" as used in this statute is defined as:

"The incorporation of physician supervision to the certified registered nurse practitioner's performance of medical acts in the following ways:

(i) Immediate availability of a licensed physician through direct communications or by radio, telephone or telecommunications.
(ii) A predetermined plan for emergency services which has been jointly developed by the supervising physician and the certified registered nurse practitioner.
(iii) A physician available on a regularly scheduled basis for:
    (a) Referrals.
    (b) Review of the standards of medical practice incorporating consultation and chart review.
    (c) Establishing and updating standing orders, drug and other medical protocols within the practice setting.
    (d) Periodic updating in medical diagnosis and therapeutics.
    (e) Cosigning records when necessary to document accountability by both parties."

Based on this definition of medical direction, one might think that Pennsylvania is a supervision state. On the other hand, Pennsylvania also seems like a collaboration state in that the regulations require the NP to work in collaboration with a licensed physician. The inclusion of both collaboration and supervision language makes Pennsylvania a good example of a combination state. Like other states highlighted in this memorandum, Pennsylvania's direction requirement specifically requires that a physician be available, either in person or through telecommunication, for consultation. In addition, the regulations also require that the supervising physician and NP develop a plan for emergency services (Pa. Code. tit. 49, § 21.251, LEXIS, current through Apr. 15, 2006). Finally, the physician must also be available to receive referrals from the NP; review the standards of medical practice, including consultation and chart review; establish and update drug and medical protocols; periodically update diagnosis and therapeutic techniques; and cosign records when appropriate (Pa. Code. tit. 49, § 21.251, LEXIS, current through Apr. 15, 2006).

This language is very similar to the other prescriptive authority statutes and supports the conclusion of this memorandum, which is that the title language of a state's physician involvement/prescriptive authority statute does not provide an adequate basis for making a generalization about the level of physician involvement required in that state. Whether a state uses collaboration, supervision, delegation, or some combination of the three descriptive designations has little practical impact. The true extent of physician involvement can only be determined by examining how each state interprets this language.

STEP 3—SECTION C: INSURANCE CARRIERS BY STATE

Locate your state and identify some of your major insurance carriers.

STEP 4—SECTION D: INSURANCE CARRIERS' CREDENTIALING CONTACT INFORMATION

For more information about health insurance companies' credentialing, please visit www.nncc.us.

CAQH

What Is the CAQH?

The Council for Affordable Health Care (CAQH) and various health plans developed a universal credentialing database with a single application for use by participating health plans and hospitals. With CAQH, practitioners use a standard application to submit one application, to one source, and update it on a quarterly basis to meet the needs of all of the health plans and hospitals that participate.

How Do I Enroll With CAQH?

Apply with a participating insurance plan and advise them that you want a CAQH application. The insurance carrier then gives CAQH your name and their provider number. CAQH will then mail you a welcome package with a

CAQH provider number. Once you receive the welcome package, go online to the CAQH website to create a user name and password and fill out the uniform application. At this point, all future insurance carriers that participate can reference this one application.

Contact Information

To find an updated list of participating plans or to get more information, go to http://caqh.org/participatingorgs.php or call 202.861.1492.

STEP 5—APPLICATION FOLLOW-UP

Once your application request has been made to the insurance company, the following general process will occur (although there may be some differences in flow with some companies):

Your initial request for an application is just that—a request for, not an actual, application. Your request may be made with the insurance company itself or through CAQH. When this request reaches the company's credentialing department, that department confirms the company's need for that provider type in that particular area in a "needs database." If the need is there, you will then be contacted with an application, and the process will continue. If there is no need, the company will regretfully deny your request.

This needs database is populated by the provider business unit (or provider contracting). If they do not include NPs in the database as needed or accepted in the area, then the credentialing department cannot move forward with the application process.

STEP 6—NNCC FOLLOW-UP

Please contact NNCC with any problems or concerns along the way. Once you are notified of your acceptance or rejection from the network, we would like to know. If necessary, we want to assist in educating these companies on the law and hopefully changing their business decisions.

A Possible Temporary Solution: Contracting as a Facility

Some managed care organizations (MCOs) have contracted with retail clinics as facilities. The retail clinic receives a flat fee per encounter. The amount of the flat fee depends on the complexity of the case, whether the patient is existing or new, and whether a vaccine was administered or not. When the MCO contracts with a facility, there is no credentialing process, and no site visits are required. NOTE: They are not contracting with the NPs individually as PCPs, and therefore no payment is made to the NP directly; the NP is paid by the facility.

Concerns

When NPs are not contracted as PCPs:

- A patient in a health maintenance organization (HMO) who needs to select a PCP cannot designate the facility as the PCP. If a referral is needed to a specialist, this could be a potential liability for the NP if he or she cannot easily refer the patient. We understand that the HMO will recognize referral by your corroborating physician.
- Patients could face additional difficulties using health plans that require referrals if the MCO system does not have a PCP listed.
- The patient has to pay the specialist co-pay when using the clinic, which can be significantly higher than the PCP co-pay.
- For the MCO, if the facility is in a capitated area (a predetermined monthly fee is paid to the patient's preselected PCP, regardless of the number of visits made by the patient), then there is potential for double payment by the MCO (to the PCP and the clinic).

Benefits

- If the facility is in a noncapitated market (fee-for-service payments), this could give the clinic some money for services via the flat fee per encounter (without the double payment concern for the MCO). If the clinic wanted to, they *could* be able to waive the specialist co-pay for their patients. While this might not be the best long-term solution, it would be a means of obtaining some financial reimbursement for the care the clinic provided.

INDEX